Pediatric and Adolescent Concussion

Jennifer Niskala Apps · Kevin D. Walter
Editors

Pediatric and Adolescent Concussion

Diagnosis, Management and Outcomes

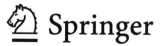 Springer

Editors
Jennifer Niskala Apps
Department of Psychiatry
and Behavioral Medicine
Medical College of Wisconsin

Children's Hospital of Wisconsin
Milwaukee, WI, USA
japps@chw.org

Kevin D. Walter
Departments of Orthopaedics
and Pediatrics
Medical College of Wisconsin

Children's Hospital of Wisconsin
Milwaukee, WI, USA
kwalter@chw.org

ISBN 978-0-387-89544-4   e-ISBN 978-0-387-89545-1
DOI 10.1007/978-0-387-89545-1
Springer New York Dordrecht Heidelberg London

Library of Congress Control Number: 2011941868

Printed on acid-free paper

Springer is part of Springer Science+Business Media (www.springer.com)

Preface

As health care providers for children, we are dedicated to giving kids of all ages the best care possible. During training, we each developed a strong interest in concussion-related concerns which peaked while treating the increasing number of children presenting in our individual practices. Upon collaborating to develop a formal clinic to attempt to best treat these children, the focus on concussion diagnosis and treatment became a passion. As with many aspects of pediatric care, not enough focused information is available to help the child and adolescent practitioner best serve this population. Through interaction with a number of other professionals, from teachers and athletic trainers to parents to pediatricians, we felt limited in our ability to provide resources and education. Thus, the idea for this book was born.

It is difficult to be both comprehensive and all-inclusive in a rapidly expanding field. This is reflected even in the title of our book, which focuses on "concussion." Use of this term is debated, with some of the authors in this book (see Chap. 2 for example) pointing out that mild traumatic brain injury (mTBI) could be considered a more appropriate term. However, we have chosen to include a wide number of opinions in this book, focusing on the use of more common terms to allow for a wide readership base. We would like this book to be useful for caregivers with significantly different backgrounds. As a result, the reader will likely note a variation in opinions and perspectives, but we felt it was important for all to be represented. As editors, we purposely chose our contributing authors in an attempt to provide the most up-to-date and expansive views across the myriad of professional fields. We have allowed these authors to use their own voices to communicate important aspects of this topic. We hope that in doing so, we have represented the complexity of this rapidly developing and expanding field, while also giving the reader a strong foundation in fact and knowledge about the assessment, diagnosis, management, recovery, and prevention of these injuries.

Each chapter is intended to stand alone and work in coordination with the book as a whole. As a reader, you may wish to read the work from beginning to end, in which case we hope you will find the experience vastly educational. However, by contrast and particularly depending on your own level of expertise with this injury, you may find it just as useful to read chapters individually. For enjoyment, you could start your journey with the case story presented at the end of Chapter 12.

Most of all, we intend to help bring a voice to this massively important injury in childhood and adolescence. Too many children are suffering needlessly during their recovery process because too many adults who care for them are not adequately educated about concussion and how to recognize and treat it. We hope that this work will improve the knowledge base available for all those who care for kids.

Milwaukee, WI, USA   Jennifer Niskala Apps
Milwaukee, WI, USA   Kevin D. Walter

Acknowledgements

Our deepest thanks to Robert Newby, PhD, ABPP. The quality of this work improved exponentially by your involvement. For all your guidance, mentorship and honesty, we are truly thankful.

I dedicate this work to my family – my husband for all of his never-ending support and belief in me, not to mention his ability to pique my competitive, sports-driven nature; and my children. Being a parent, I have learned the true value and motivation of life.

Jennifer Niskala Apps PhD

We would like to thank all of our authors for their hard work. It is a pleasure to be involved in a project with people we hold in such high regard.

I dedicate this work to my wife Katie, without her support and love I could not accomplish my goals. I also dedicate this to Abby, Claire and Ryan, you are all of my future hopes and dreams.

Kevin D. Walter, MD

Contents

Part III   Additional Issues in Pediatric Concussion

Abbreviations

AAP	American Academy of Pediatrics
ACE	Acute Concussion Evaluation
ACRM	American Congress of Rehabilitation Medicine
ADL	Activities of Daily Living
APOE4	Apolipoprotein E Allele 4
ANAM	Automated Neuropsychological Assessment Metrics
ATP	Adenosine Triphosphate
BASC	Behavior Assessment System for Children
BDNF	Brain-Derived Neurotrophic Factor
BESS	Balance-Error Scoring System
BOLD	Blood Oxygen Level Dependent
BRC	Brain Reserve Capacity
CBCL	Child Behavior Checklist
CDC	Centers for Disease Control and Prevention
CIS	Concussion in Sport
CISG	Concussion in Sport Group
CNS	Central Nervous System
CT	Computed Tomography
CTP	Cleaved Tau Protein
DAI	Diffuse Axonal Injury
DLPFC	Dorsolateral Prefrontal Cortex/Cortical
DSM-IV	Diagnostic and Statistical Manual of Mental Disorders, Fourth Edition
DTI	Diffusion Tensor Imaging
EAA	Excitatory Neurotransmitters
ED	Emergency Department
EMS	Emergency Medical Services
FA	Fractional Anisotropy
fMRI	Functional MRI
g	Grams
GCS	Glasgow Coma Scale
GP	Game Positions

HS RIO	High School Reporting Information Online
ICD-10	International Statistical Classification of Diseases and Related Health Problems – 10th revision
ImPACT	Immediate Post-Concussion Assessment and Cognitive Testing
INS	Interpersonal Negotiation Strategies
ISS	Injury Surveillance System
LOC	Loss of Consciousness
m/s	Meters per Second
MPH	Miles per Hour
MRA	Magnetic Resonance Angiography
MRI	Magnetic Resonance Imaging
MRS	Magnetic Resonance Spectroscopy
ms	Millisecond
MSI	Magnetic Source Imaging
mTBI	Mild Traumatic Brain Injury
N	Newtons
NATA	National Athletic Trainers Association
NCAA	National Collegiate Athletic Association
NFHS	National Federation for State High School Associations
NFL	National Football League
NOCSAE	National Operating Committee on Standards for Athletic Equipment
NSE	Neuron Specific Enolase
OAS	Overt Aggression Scale
PCD	Post-Concussion Disorder
PCS	Post-Concussion Syndrome
PCSI	Post-Concussion Symptom Inventory
PET	Positron Emission Tomography
PPCS	Persistent Post-Concussive Syndrome
PTA	Post-Traumatic Amnesia
SAC	Standardized Assessment of Concussion
SCAT	Sport Concussion Assessment Tool
SCAT2	Sport Concussion Assessment Tool – Second Edition
SES	Socio-Economic Status
SI	Severity Index
SPECT	Single Photon Emission Computed Tomography
SSRI	Selective Serotonin Reuptake Inhibitor
TBI	Traumatic Brain Injury
TMJ	Temporomandibular Joint
VABS	Vineland Adaptive Behavior Scales
WHO	World Health Organization

Contributors

Jennifer Niskala Apps, PhD Associate Professor, Department of Psychiatry and Behavioral Medicine, Medical College of Wisconsin

Pediatric Neuropsychologist, Children's Hospital of Wisconsin, Milwaukee, WI, USA

David T. Bernhardt, MD Professor, Department of Pediatrics, Orthopedics and Rehabilitation, University of Wisconsin School of Medicine and Public Health, Madison, WI, USA

Doug Bodin, PhD, ABPP/CN Pediatric Neuropsychologist, Assistant Clinical Professor of Pediatrics, Nationwide Children's Hospital, The Ohio State University, Columbus, OH, USA

Susannah M. Briskin, MD Associate Professor of Pediatrics, Co-Director of Primary Care Sports Medicine Fellowship, Rainbow Babies and Children's Hospital, University Hospitals Case Medical Center, Cleveland, OH, USA

Monique S. Burton, MD, FAAP Interim Chief, Sports Medicine Program, Seattle Children's Hospital, Clinical Assistant Professor, Department of Pediatrics and Orthopedics and Sports Medicine, University of Washington, Seattle, WA, USA

Brianne Butcher, PhD Postdoctoral Resident in Clinical Neuropsychology, Children's Medical Center of Dallas, Dallas, TX, USA

Katherine S. Dahab, MD Primary Care Sports Medicine Fellow, University of Wisconsin, Milwaukee, WI, USA

Rebecca A. Demorest, MD, FAAP Associate Medical Director, Pediatric and Young Adult Sports Medicine, Children's Hospital & Research Center Oakland, Oakland, CA, USA

Jason S. Doescher, MD Pediatric Neurology and Epilepsy,
Minnesota Epilepsy Group, P.A.
Children's Hospital and Clinics of Minnesota, Saint Paul, MN, USA

Gerard A. Gioia, PhD Chief, Division of Pediatric Neuropsychology, Director
Safe Concussion Outcome Recovery and Education (SCORE) Program
Associate Professor, Departments of Pediatric and Psychiatry and Behavioral
Sciences, George Washington University of Medicine, Washington, DC, USA

Mark E. Halstead, MD, FAAP Assistant Professor, Department of Pediatrics
and Orthopedics, Washington University School of Medicine, Director,
Sports Concussion Clinic, St. Louis, MO, USA

Nathan E. Kegel, PhD Neuropsychology Fellow, University of Pittsburgh
Medical Center, Sports Medicine Concussion Program, Pittsburgh, PA, USA

Karl Klamar, MD, FAAPM&R Clinical Assistant Professor, Pediatric
Rehabilitation Medicine, Nationwide Children's Hospital, Physical Medicine
and Rehabilitation, Ohio State University Medical Center, Columbus, OH, USA

Mark R. Lovell, PhD, FACPN Professor and Director, University of Pittsburgh
Medical Center, Sports Medicine Concussion Program, Pittsburgh, PA, USA

Teri Metcalf McCambridge, MD Associate Professor of Pediatrics,
Director of Sports Medicine Division, Cincinnati Children's Hospital Medical
Center, Cincinnati, OH, USA

Michael McCrea, PhD, ABPP Director of Brain Injury Research, Departments of
Neurosurgery and Neurology, Medical College of Wisconsin, Milwaukee, WI, USA

Mathew R. Powell, PhD, ABPP Neuropsychology Department,
Minocqua Behavioral Health, Marshfield Clinic, Minocqua, WI, USA

Jonathan E. Romain, PhD, ABPP/CN Department of Psychiatry
and Behavioral Medicine, Children's Hospital of Wisconsin, Milwaukee, WI, USA

Maegan D.S. Sady, PhD Division of Pediatric Neuropsychology, Children's
National Medical Center, Washington, DC, USA

Alice Ann Spurgin, BA Doctoral Candidate in Clinical Psychology,
Neuropsychology Intern, Children's Medical Center of Dallas, University of Texas
Southwestern Medical Center, Dallas, TX, USA

Peter L. Stavinoha, PhD, ABPP Director of Neuropsychology, Professor of
Psychology, Children's Medical Center of Dallas, University of Texas
Southwestern Medical Center, Dallas, TX, USA

Danny G. Thomas, MD, MPH Assistant Professor of Pediatrics
Emergency Medicine, Medical College of Wisconsin, Milwaukee, WI, USA

Amy E. Valasek, MD Assistant Professor, Department of Orthopedics, Pediatric Division, Johns Hopkins Hospital, White Marsh, MD, USA

Christopher G. Vaughan, PsyD Division of Pediatric Neuropsychology, Children's National Medical Center

Assistant Professor, Departments of Pediatrics and Psychiatry and Behavioral Sciences, George Washington University School of Medicine, Washington, DC, USA

Kevin D. Walter, MD, FAAP Assistant Professor, Departments of Orthopaedics and Pediatrics, Medical College of Wisconsin

Program Director, Pediatric and Adolescent Sports Medicine, Children's Hospital of Wisconsin, Milwaukee, WI, USA

Amanda K. Weiss Kelly, MD Associate Professor of Pediatrics, Co-Director of Primary Care Sports Medicine Fellowship, Rainbow Babies and Children's Hospital, University Hospitals Case Medical Center, Cleveland, OH, USA

Keith Owen Yeates, PhD, ABPP/CN Chief, Department of Psychology, Professor Department of Pediatrics, Director Center for Biobehavioral Health, Nationwide Children's Hospital, The Ohio State University, The Research Institute at Nationwide Children's Hospital, Columbus, OH, USA

Part I
Definitions and Causes of Concussion

Chapter 1
Historical Perspectives on Concussion

Mark E. Halstead

1.1 Introduction

The understanding of concussions has evolved substantially over time, both over the history of medicine and specifically during the past decade. From an initial description over a thousand years ago of a concussion as more of a symptom of head injury to the current concept of a functional rather than a structural brain injury, knowledge of the condition continues to expand. Medical knowledge is likely still in its infancy with regard to truly understanding a concussion and all its nuances. This chapter serves to describe the evolution of understanding of concussion, as well as some history of the use of protective devices intended to reduce the likelihood of a concussive events during athletics.

1.2 Early Concepts of Concussive Events

Early accounts of medical descriptions of concussive injury are sparse. Most descriptions were from ancient literature, such as Homer's epics in the second millennium BC, rather than physicians. Homer described symptoms that Hector experienced in a battle for Troy, including weakness of the knees and vision clouding, which rapidly recovered allowing him to continue battling (Wrightson 2000). Hippocrates described clinical symptoms of head injuries, including the account of an 11-year-old boy kicked in the head by a horse, but nothing specific to a concussive event. More complicated injuries were managed by probing the wound with a

M.E. Halstead (✉)
Department of Pediatrics and Orthopedics, Washington University School of Medicine,
Sports Concussion Clinic, St. Louis, MO, USA
e-mail: halsteadm@wustl.edu

J.N. Apps and K.D. Walter (eds.), *Pediatric and Adolescent Concussion:*
Diagnosis, Management and Outcomes, DOI 10.1007/978-0-387-89545-1_1,
© Springer Science+Business Media, LLC 2012

metal object to determine if a skull fracture had occurred. If no skull fracture was found, the wound would then be trephined with the expectation that humors would be released or the skull tightness could be slackened to help treat the head injury (Hippocrates 1849).

In 900 AD, the Arabic physician Rhazes first described a concussion as a separate entity, along the line of current thinking of a transient state of abnormal physiology in the brain. In 1280 AD, Lanfrancus introduced a similar concept as Rhazes focusing on the commotio (shaking) of the brain that would produce the clinical picture of concussion. Lanfrancus described the symptoms as being a result of transient paralysis of cerebral function (McHenry 1969). Early in the fourteenth century, Guy de Chauliac made note of particularly good outcomes from concussions as opposed to an injury resulting in a skull fracture.

In the sixteenth century, descriptions of concussions fitting with modern day concepts were beginning. Berengario da Carpi described the injury as being caused by the brain tissue striking the skull without any readily apparent external signs of head injury (Putti 1937). Similar to Rhazes, da Carpi describes this phenomenon as a "succusio" or shaking of the brain. Pare wrote an entire chapter about concussions in his book, which was fairly uncommon at that time, calling them a disorder of the brain movement with brain swelling and hemorrhage (Pare 1579). In 1573, Coiter documented many symptoms of concussion, including memory impairment, faltering of speech, poor judgment, and difficulty with understanding (Coiter 1573).

With the development of the microscope in the early seventeenth century, more physiologic analysis of the injury began. Concussions were considered to be a separate injury rather than a symptom of overall head injury. Recovery was noted to typically occur over a short period of time with symptoms such as photophobia, tinnitus, and giddiness (McCrory and Berkovic 2001). Thomas Kirkland noted in the late eighteenth century that concussions were not structural injuries, and if bleeding in the brain occurred it would be a later phenomenon (Kirkland 1792). In 1705, Littre described this phenomenon in a case report of a young man that instantly died after diving head first into a wall while attempting to evade his execution. No lesions were found on the autopsy but it was felt that death occurred through an emptying of the cortical blood vessels (Littre 1705).

In 1830, John Abernathy developed a more extensive description of symptoms of a concussion, such as one not being in a normal state of health, that others had previous felt were insignificant to include in their discussion (Abernathy 1830). Sir John Erichsen in 1853, in his "The Science and Art of Surgery," defined concussion as an impairment of consciousness lasting for minutes to hours, with symptoms of confusion and giddiness lasting for a few days after. Most individuals were felt to recover fully, but some would not be able to resume their regular occupation due to impairment of mental function (Erichsen 1895).

Among the first descriptions of lingering symptoms in some patients, perhaps as a postconcussive syndrome, were those made by John Hilton in 1863 in his "Lectures on Rest and Pain" (Hilton 1877). For the next hundred years, postconcussive symptoms were often felt to be due to malingering or a form of neurosis. In 1927, Osnato and Giliberti described 100 cases of concussion and felt that if symptoms did not recover completely then degeneration in the brain occurred (Onsanto and Giliberti 1927). Since symptoms that did not resolve could be similar to encephalitis, these authors coined the term traumatic encephalitis. Romanis and Mitchiner observed in the 1930s that most cases recovered within 2 weeks, which is consistent with current thinking (Romanis and Mitchiner 1934). Patients with postconcussive symptoms longer than 2 weeks were labeled as having traumatic neurasthenia. In 1961, Henry Miller wrote that persistent symptoms were rare when no compensation claims were pending, as in typical sports injury situations (Miller 1961). He proposed that injury severity was felt to be inversely related to the duration of coma and amnesia. This was in direct contrast of Sir Charles Symonds who, in 1960, described evidence of lasting symptoms and felt these were a direct result of neuronal injury (Symonds 1962).

The first specification of long-term sequelae of repeated concussions in sports was the "Punch Drunk" syndrome described by Martland in 1928. Early symptoms were described as shuffling of the feet or difficulty moving the feet, occasionally forcing a boxer into retirement and/or even commitment to an asylum. This was the first description of Parkinsonian-like symptoms that these athletes could develop (Martland 1928). In 1934, Parker coined the term traumatic encephalopathy for these cases of boxers with the "Punch Drunk" syndrome. In one of three cases described, there were also accounts of physical exertion exacerbating the boxers' symptoms (Parker 1934).

Reginald Kelly felt that prolonged concussion symptoms were due to a failure to acknowledge and treat the problem. He believed that patients who suffered from postconcussive symptoms had an iatrogenic etiology due to the doctors' failure to treat it (Kelly 1981).

Denny-Brown and Russell looked at the mechanism of concussion with studies on cats in the 1940s. Injuries were felt to be produced through acceleration–deceleration and rotational shear forces to the brain (Denny-Brown and Russell 1941). Further studies with rats in the 1980s and 1990s found that damage at the cellular level produced metabolic abnormalities in the brain, leading to the "metabolic crisis" theory in describing concussions (Foda and Marmorou 1994). Injuries were felt to be produced through acceleration–deceleration and rotational shear forces to the brain. Further studies with rats in the 1980s found that damage at the cellular level produced the metabolic abnormalities (Foda and Marmorou 1994).

1.3 Initial Neuropsychological Research on Sport-Related Concussion

Early concepts of the neurocognitive issues were established by Ruesch in the 1940s, who demonstrated reduced performance in tests of speed of thinking and fatigability in concussed patients (Ruesch and Bowman 1945). These deficits were found to improve over a few weeks. In 1958, Dencker and Lofving described head injuries in twins where the concussed twin had a more difficult time with complex tasks than the nonconcussed twin (Dencker and Lofving 1958). In 1974, Lidvall described patients who underwent a large battery of cognitive and behavioral tests, in addition to vestibular studies and EEGs, and found no abnormalities in patients with postconcussive syndrome. It was felt that their symptoms must be related to poor motivation or depression rather than concussive symptoms, further sparking the debate on the actual cause of postconcussive symptoms (Lidvall et al. 1974). The more recent burgeoning neuropsychological contribution to this research is beyond the scope of this historical review and is noted in many of the subsequent chapters of this book.

1.4 Modern Guidelines on Sports-Related Concussion

In 2001, the first International Symposia on Concussion in Sport was held in Vienna, Austria. This was organized by the Federation Internationale de Football, the International Olympic Committee and the International Ice Hockey Federation. Individuals who were considered to be experts in the field of sport-related concussions convened to come up with new guidelines and recommendations on the diagnosis and management of head injuries in sports (Aubry et al. 2002). Further meetings in Prague in 2004 and Zurich in 2008 have refined these recommendations which now constitute the framework for most decision-making processes in sport-related concussion. In September 2010, the American Academy of Pediatrics published a clinical report on sport-related concussions in children and adolescents, becoming the first major group to offer guidelines specific to the pediatric population (Halstead et al. 2010).

1.5 History of Protective Equipment

In response to several deaths related to head injuries sustained in football, the first helmets, made primarily of leather, were used in an Army–Navy game in 1893. The National Collegiate Athletic Association (NCAA) made helmets mandatory in football in 1939 with the National Football League (NFL) following in 1940. The addition of a single bar face mask was made in 1951, and the first double bar face mask was used in 1958. Safety standards were developed in 1973 by the National Operating Committee on Standards for Athletic Equipment (NOCSAE), 4 years after its founding. These standards were comprised using an apparatus with a helmeted head model which would be subsequently dropped in various directions, known as the "drop test." In 1975, a rule against spear tackling was created after a large number of head and neck injuries were seen when players would lead with their helmet to initiate a tackle, effectively making the helmet a weapon (Levy et al. 2004).

In addition to the traditional helmet, now used in multiple sports and occupations with a high risk of head injury, other equipment has been utilized to potentially reduce the risk of concussion. Mouth guards are often debated as offering a possible protective effect from concussion. Boxing was the first sport to use mouth guards in the late nineteenth century. Materials used in these early mouth guards included cotton, tape, sponges or small pieces of wood. As one can imagine, there were case reports of these materials becoming dislodged and entering the larynx. In the 1890s, Woolf Krause, a dentist from London, started using a rubber-like resin strip over the boxers' maxillary incisors prior to entering the ring (Knapik et al. 2007). Following an endorsement from the American Dental Association, football adopted the use of mouth guards in 1960. This was also in response to the high rate of dental injuries in football, ranging from 23 to 54% of all football injuries, in the 1940s and 1950s. High school and junior college football adopted mouth guard use in 1962. The NCAA mandated mouth guard use in 1973 for football, but also now requires them in ice hockey, lacrosse, and field hockey. Although mouth guard use has been very effective in reducing the likelihood of dental trauma, there has not been convincing evidence as to their effectiveness in reducing concussions (Knapik et al. 2007).

1.6 Summary

Since ancient times, the understanding of concussions has evolved dramatically along with medical science. Over the past century, significant advancements occurred furthering this understanding at a biochemical level. The use of protective equipment to potentially reduce the effects of sport-related concussion has also advanced during this time. As research continues, we can only expect to better our skills in the diagnosis and management of concussions, adding to the rich history of this fascinating injury.

1.7 Key Points

Early understanding of a concussion focused more on the injury as a symptom, rather than a unique injury.

By the eighteenth century, modern theories and thinking of concussion as a distinct injury had developed.

As recently as the early twentieth century, patients with postconcussive symptoms were thought of as malingerers.

Early knowledge of the long-term sequelae of concussions came from boxers.

References

Abernathy, J. (1830). *On injuries of the head. Surgical and physiological works* (Vol. 2). London: Longman, Ress, Orme, Brown and Green.

Aubry, M., Cantu, R., Dvorak, J., Grat-Baumann, T., Johnston, K., Kelly, J., et al. (2002). Summary and agreement statement of the first international conference on concussion in sport, Vienna 2001. *British Journal of Sports Medicine, 36*, 6–10.

Coiter, V. (1573). Externarum et internarum principalium humani corporis partiumtabulae atque anatomicae exerctitationes observationesque variae. Noribergae: T Gerlatzeni.

Dencker, S., & Lofving, B. (1958). A psychometric study of identical twins discordant for closed head injury. *Acta Psychiatrica et Neurologica Scandinavica Supplementum, 122*, 1–50.

Denny-Brown, D., & Russell, W. (1941). Experimental cerebral concussion. *Brain, 54*, 93–164.

Erichsen, J. (1895). *The science and art of surgery* (10th ed.). London: Longmans Green.

Foda, M., & Marmorou, A. (1994). A new model of diffuse brain injury in rats. Part II: morphological characterization. *Journal of Neurosurgery, 80*, 301–313.

Halstead, M., Walter, K., Council on Sports Medicine and Fitness. (2010). Sport-related concussion in children and adolescents. *Pediatrics, 126*, 597–615.

Hilton, J. (1877). *On rest and pain* (2nd ed.). London: George Bell.

Hippocrates. (1849). *The genuine works of Hippocrates*. London: The Syndenham Society.

Kelly, R. (1981). The post-traumatic syndrome. *Journal of Royal Society of Medicine, 74*, 242–244.

Kirkland, T. (1792). *A commentary on apoplectic and paralytic affections and on diseases connected with the subject*. London: William Dawson.

Knapik, J., Marshall, S., Lee, R., Darakjzy, SS., Jones, SB., Mitchener, TA., et al. (2007). Mouthguards in sport activities: history, physical properties and injury prevention effectiveness. *Sports Medicine, 37*, 117–144.

Levy, M., Ozgur, B., Berry, C., Aryan, HE., Apuzzo, ML., et al. (2004). Birth and evolution of the football helmet. *Neurosurgery, 55*, 656–662.

Lidvall, H., Linderoth, B., & Norlin, B. (1974). Causes of the post-concussional syndrome. *Acta Neurologica Scandinavica Supplementum, 56*, 3–144.

Littre, M. (1705). *Histoire de L'Academie Royale des Sciences*. Paris: L'Academie Royale des Sciences.

Martland, H. (1928). Punch Drunk. *Journal of American Medical Association, 91*, 1103–1107.

McCrory, P., & Berkovic, S. (2001). Concussion: the history of clinical and pathophysiological concepts and misconceptions. *Neurology, 57*, 2283–2289.

McHenry, L. (1969). *Garrison's history of neurology*. Springfield: Charles C Thomas.

Miller, H. (1961). Accident neurosis. *British Medical Journal, 1*(919–925), 992–998.

Onsanto, M., & Giliberti, V. (1927). Postconcussion neurosis – traumatic encephalitis. *Archives of Neurology and Psychiatry, 18*, 181–211.

Pare, A. (1579). *The works of that famous chirurgion Ambrose Parey*. London: Cotes and Young.

Parker, H. (1934). Traumatic encephalopathy of professional pugilists. *Journal of Neurology and Psychopathology, s1–15*, 20–28.

Putti, V. (1937). *Berengario da Carpi, saggio biografico c bibliographico*. Bologna: L Capelli.

Romanis, W., & Mitchiner, P. (1934). *The science and practice of surgery*, Vol 2, 5th edn. Philadelphia: Lea and Febiger.

Ruesch, J., & Bowman, K. (1945). Prolonged post-traumatic syndromes following head injury. *American Journal of Psychiatry, 102*, 145–163.

Symonds, C. (1962). Concussion and its sequelae. *Lancet, 1*, 1–5.

Wrightson, P. (2000). The development of a concept of mild head injury. *Journal of Clinical Neuroscience, 7*, 384–388.

Chapter 2
Definition and Classification of Concussion

Doug Bodin, Keith Owen Yeates, and Karl Klamar

2.1 Introduction

Traumatic brain injury (TBI) is a leading cause of hospitalization and death among children and adolescents and therefore represents a major public health problem (Langlois et al. 2006). Recent estimates of pediatric TBI suggest an annual incidence of 475,000 cases for children ages 0 to 14 (Langlois et al. 2006). However, most studies of TBI prevalence (i.e., all cases) and incidence (i.e., new cases) only include injuries associated with hospitalization resulting in fewer documented cases of milder forms of TBI such as concussions (Yeates 2010). Two relatively recent population based studies in Canada have documented estimated prevalence rates for pediatric concussion at 200 per 100,000 (Gordon et al. 2006) and 135 per 100,000 (Willer et al. 2004). However, these two studies are likely underestimates of the true prevalence of concussion, as the Gordon et al. (2006) study relied on retrospective report by parents of concussion that limited daily activity, and the Willer et al. (2004) study relied on narrative descriptions made by school staff not trained in recognizing the symptoms of concussion. Data from the US Centers for Disease Control and Prevention (CDC, Langlois et al. 2006) suggest that the prevalence rate for mild TBI in children is higher than these two studies when based on emergency department visits.

D. Bodin (✉)
Nationwide Children's Hospital, The Ohio State University, Columbus, OH, USA
e-mail: doug.bodin@NationwideChildrens.org

K.O. Yeates
Department of Psychology, Professor Department of Pediatrics, Director Center
for Biobehavioral Health, Nationwide Children's Hospital, The Ohio State University,
The Research Institute at Nationwide Children's Hospital, Columbus, OH, USA

K. Klamar
Pediatric Rehabilitation Medicine, Nationwide Children's Hospital,
Physical Medicine and Rehabilitation, Ohio State University Medical Center,
Columbus, OH, USA

J.N. Apps and K.D. Walter (eds.), *Pediatric and Adolescent Concussion:*
Diagnosis, Management and Outcomes, DOI 10.1007/978-0-387-89545-1_2,
© Springer Science+Business Media, LLC 2012

In the past decade, increased attention has been given to milder forms of TBI, such as concussion. The increased recognition and diagnosis of concussion has occurred largely in the area of sports medicine. In fact, over 50% of pediatric concussions are estimated to occur in the context of sports participation (Gordon et al. 2006). Despite this increased recognition, and resulting scientific and professional literature regarding concussions, a substantial lack of agreement persists regarding the definition and classification of concussions. The goal of this chapter is to provide a review of the definition and classification of concussions, with special attention to pediatric populations, as well as to review several nosological issues that arise during the course of both clinical and research work.

2.2 Definitions of Relevant Terms

The term "concussion" is not well defined in either clinical or research contexts, leading to confusion among patients, families, and even many health providers regarding the importance of this diagnosis. As a diagnosis, concussion is often used interchangeably with terms such as mild traumatic brain injury (mTBI), minor closed head injury, and mild closed head injury. Concussion is more often used in the sports medicine community, whereas mTBI is sometimes the preferred term in other medical specialties (Tator 2009). Many authors use the term "concussion" in reference to head injuries that result in only transient neurological deficits. Others have argued that the term concussion should be used to place an emphasis on impaired functional status following a head trauma, whereas mild head injury should be used to place an emphasis on subsequent pathophysiology (Anderson et al. 2006).

Based on a 2010 study, DeMatteo found that using the term concussion when a patient is admitted to the hospital may unintentionally communicate to parents that a "brain injury" did not occur, resulting in less than adequate follow-up with appropriate healthcare providers. Therefore, recommendations were made for using "mTBI" instead of "concussion" (DeMatteo et al. 2010). An alternative perspective is that concussion is a variant of mTBI and that the term "minimal head injury" be used in place of "concussion" to denote an injury that is not accompanied by any loss of consciousness (LOC) and yields a Glasgow Coma Scale (GCS; Teasdale and Jennett 1974) score of 15; by contrast, "mild head injury" would denote a injury with brief LOC and GCS of 14–15 (Falk et al. 2005). For the purpose of this chapter, the term "concussion" will be used interchangeably with "mTBI." Other chapters in this work will also reflect these differences in the use of terminology.

Several organizations have attempted to provide a definition for concussion or mTBI; however, a consensus has yet to emerge. One of the earliest attempts at a definition was made in 1966 by the Congress of Neurological Surgeons (1966). In that definition, concussion was defined as "a clinical syndrome characterized by immediate and transient impairment of neural functions, such as alteration of consciousness, disturbance of vision, equilibrium, etc. due to mechanical forces."

Table 2.1 Definitional criteria for concussion/mTBI

	LOC	PTA	Mental status	Neurological signs
ACRM	≤30 min	≤24 h	Any alteration in mental status at time of injury	May or may not be transient
AAP	≤1 min	Not specified	Normal mental status at time of initial evaluation	None at exam, but may have seizures or other signs immediately following injury
WHO	≤30 min	≤24 h	Confusion and disorientation	Transient neurological abnormalities

LOC Loss of consciousness, *PTA* posttraumatic amnesia, *ACRM* American Congress of Rehabilitation Medicine, *WHO* World Health Organization, *AAP* American Academy of Pediatrics

The American Congress of Rehabilitation Medicine (ACRM; Mild Traumatic Brain Injury Committee 1993) developed the following definition for mTBI:

> "A traumatically induced disruption of brain function, as manifested by at least one of the following: any LOC, any loss of memory for events immediately before or after the accident, any alteration in mental state at the time of the accident, and focal neurological deficit(s) that may or may not be transient; but where the severity of the injury does not exceed the following: LOC of approximately 30 min or less, after 30 min an initial GDS score of 13–15, and posttraumatic amnesia (PTA) not greater than 24 h."

The American Academy of Pediatrics' definition of minor closed head injury includes the following criteria: normal mental status at the initial examination, no abnormal or focal neurological findings, no physical evidence of skull fracture, LOC of less than 1 min; and can have seizures, emesis, headache, and lethargy immediately after the injury (AAP; Committee on Quality Improvement and Pediatrics 1999). More recently, the World Health Organization (WHO) has proffered a definition similar to that of ACRM (Carroll et al. 2004):

> "MTBI is an acute brain injury resulting from mechanical energy to the head from external physical forces. Operational criteria for clinical identification include (1) 1 or more of the following: confusion or disorientation, LOC for 30 min or less, posttraumatic amnesia for less than 24 h, and/or other transient neurological abnormalities such as focal signs, seizure, and intracranial lesion not requiring surgery; (2) Glasgow Coma Scale score of 13–15 after 30 min postinjury or later upon presentation for healthcare. These manifestations of MTBI must not be due to drugs, alcohol, medications, caused by other injuries or treatment for other injuries (e.g., systemic injuries, facial injuries or intubation), caused by other problems (e.g., psychological trauma, language barrier or coexisting medical conditions) or caused by penetrating craniocerebral injury".

Each of these more recent definitions places emphasis on four primary diagnostic criteria (see Table 2.1). Although similar, the three definitions do have important differences. The AAP definition is more conservative regarding length of LOC and does not specifically include length of PTA. The three definitions also differ with regard to when alterations in mental status are documented (i.e., at the time of injury in the ACRM definition vs. at the time of initial evaluation in the AAP definition). The ACRM and WHO definitions differ primarily on whether or not focal neurological signs must be transient.

The most recent consensus definition of concussion was provided by the International Symposia on Concussion in Sports (McCrory et al. 2009). This definition, often referred to as the Zurich definition, does not place an emphasis on LOC or PTA, but emphasis is placed on the functional changes that acutely follow concussion.

2.3 Classification of Concussion

Similar to the definition of concussion, much controversy exists in research and clinical contexts regarding the classification of concussions. Concussions have been classified along diagnostic and severity spectrums. Diagnostically, the International Statistical Classification of Diseases and Related Health Problems–10th revision (ICD-10; World Health Organization 1992) includes concussion as a separate code under the broader category of "intracranial injury, excluding those with skull fracture." Furthermore, the ICD-10 includes several qualifiers: with or without LOC; duration of LOC; and with or without return to preexisting levels. Based on the argument that concussions occasionally lead to lasting neurobehavioral problems (Brown et al. 1994) the Diagnostic and Statistical Manual of Mental Disorders-Fourth Edition (DSM-IV; American Psychiatric Association 1994) included research criteria for a related diagnosis termed postconcussional disorder. These criteria include a history of head trauma that has caused significant cerebral concussion, evidence from neuropsychological testing of difficulty in attention and memory, and three out of eight somatic and affective postconcussion symptoms, as well as evidence that these symptoms cause clinically significant impairment. The ICD-10 also lists postconcussion disorder, but does not require objective evidence of cognitive deficits or clinical impairment. The inconsistency between these two widely used diagnostic manuals leads to poor diagnostic agreement (Boake et al. 2004, 2005). In addition, the criteria for postconcussion syndrome in both the DSM-IV and ICD-10 have been shown to have limited specificity (Boake et al. 2005). The relevance of postconcussion syndrome has been addressed in both general (Mittenberg and Strauman 2000) and pediatric (Mittenberg et al. 1997; Yeates et al. 1999) populations.

The classification of concussion severity occurs along a broader spectrum of TBI. This broader classification is based on GSC score, length of LOC, and length of PTA (see Table 2.2) (Bodin and Yeates 2010). Because of the heterogeneity of TBI, not

Table 2.2 Ratings of TBI severity	Mild	Moderate	Severe
	GCS = 13–15	GCS = 9–12	GCS ≤ 8
	PTA ≤ 1 h	PTA = 1–24 h	PTA = >1 day
	LOC < 30 min	LOC = 30 min–24 h	LOC > 24 h

GCS Glasgow Coma Scale, *PTA* length of posttraumatic amnesia, *LOC* length of loss of consciousness

Table 2.3 Concussion grading systems

	Grade 1	Grade 2	Grade 3
Colorado Medical Society	– Confusion without amnesia – No LOC	– Confusion with amnesia – No LOC	– Any LOC
American Academy of Neurology	– Transient confusion – No LOC – Symptoms or mental status abnormalities resolve within 15 min	– Transient confusion – No LOC – Symptoms or mental status abnormalities last more than 15 min	– Any LOC
Cantu – revised	– No LOC – PTA/PCSS < 30 min	– LOC < 1 min or – PTA > 30 min < 24 h – PCSS > 30 min < 7 days	– LOC ≥1 min – PTA ≥24 h – PCSS > 7 days

all injuries fall neatly into one of these categories. For example, an injury can result in a GCS score of 6 (severe) but with an LOC of only a few hours (moderate). In recognition of the heterogeneity of TBI, numerous attempts have been made to classify concussions according to severity grading systems (Esselman and Uomoto 1995; Slobounov, 2008). For a historical review of concussion grading systems, see Slobounov (2008). The development of concussion grading systems has been primarily spurred by the sports medicine field, given the need to provide rapid side-line assessment and triage of concussed athletes (Hunt and Asplund 2010). Although no concussion grading system is universally accepted, three systems have gained widespread usage in the late 1990s based on four criteria (Slobounov 2008), although their use varies among professions (see Table 2.3).

The Colorado Medical Society's grading system classified concussions based on presence of amnesia and LOC (Colorado Medical Society 1991). A concussion resulting in confusion without amnesia and no LOC is classified as Grade 1, whereas a concussion resulting in confusion with amnesia and no LOC is Grade 2. Under this system, any LOC results in a grade 3 concussion. The American Academy of Neurology (AAN) (1997) grading system primarily distinguished concussion grades based on presence of LOC and resolution of concussion symptoms or mental status abnormalities. As in the Colorado Medical Society's grading system, the AAN system considers any concussion with an LOC to be grade 3. Grades 1 and 2 are distinguished by the resolution of acute symptoms or mental status abnormalities (i.e., within 15 min for Grade 1 and lasting longer than 15 min for Grade 2). Cantu (2001) updated his previous grading system using data from prospective studies. This grading system extended previous attempts by including length of postconcussion symptoms, based on empirical evidence that postconcussion symptoms and PTA predict poor performance on neuropsychological tests (Cantu 2001). Absence of LOC and brief PTA and postconcussion symptoms are classified as Grade 1 or mild concussion. Brief LOC, PTA up to 24 h, and postconcussion symptoms up to 7 days is classified as Grade 2 or moderate concussion. LOC longer than 1 min, PTA longer than 1 day, and postconcussion symptoms longer than 7 days is classified as a Grade 3 or severe concussion.

A more recent distinction has been made between simple and complex concussions, depending mainly on duration of postconcussive symptoms. Introduced as a result of the 2nd International Conference on Concussion in Sport held in 2004 (McCrory et al. 2005), simple concussion was defined as an injury that resolves within 10 days, whereas complex concussion was defined as an injury with persistent symptoms (i.e., more than 10 days), concussive convulsions, prolonged LOC, or prolonged cognitive impairment. This classification system has been criticized based on the fact that determining whether or not a concussion is simple or complex is a retrospective clinical judgment that does not assist practitioners in determining injury severity at the time of injury (Makdissi 2009). Indeed, the simple vs complex concussion classification system was abandoned in favor of just calling the injury a concussion at the 3rd International Conference on Concussion in Sport held in 2008 (McCrory et al. 2009), although the panel agreed that the majority of concussions show symptom resolution within 10 days (i.e., simple concussion).

2.4 Nosological Issues

Problems with the definition and classification of concussion have plagued efforts to conduct sound empirical research, resulting in controversy and misunderstanding amongst clinicians and families. No discussion of the nosology of concussion is complete without a discussion of the issues that drive these controversies.

2.4.1 Severity Ratings

The classic measure of head injury severity is the GCS, which is used to distinguish mild brain injuries, such as concussion, from more severe forms of TBI. One problem with the GCS is that it cannot readily be completed retrospectively (Ruff and Jurica 1999), because the symptoms assessed with the GCS typically are exhibited during the first few hours following the injury. This is a particular problem for mTBI, because a GCS score is often not recorded or available immediately postinjury in this population (Tator 2009; DeMatteo et al. 2010). An additional concern regarding the GCS is that it is often administered at different time points, leading to problems deciding which GCS score to use for documenting severity (Yeates 2010). Over time, duration of PTA has gained favor as a measure of TBI severity; however, PTA is not universally accepted as the best indicator of severity (Cantu 2001). For example, PTA is often assessed retrospectively and can be influenced by the patient's initial confusion around the time of injury (Esselman and Uomoto 1995). In addition, a patient's account of memories surrounding the injury can reflect what they have been told happened rather than events that they actually recall. Finally, few standardized measures of PTA are available. As mentioned previously, presence of LOC is often used to define and classify concussions. Evidence has emerged suggesting that LOC does not correlate well with concussion outcomes, leading one group to conclude that LOC not be used to measure severity of concussions (Cantu 2006). Recent research has documented a correlation between duration of postconcussion symptoms and neuropsychological test performance, resulting in increased attention to postconcussion symptoms in rating concussion severity (Cantu 2001).

Neuroimaging has also been used to assist with classifying concussions. Although traditional imaging methods may not be sensitive enough to document potential structural lesions in concussions, the use of CT scans has shown impressive sensitivity and negative predictive value in defining mTBI, meaning that CT scan can be useful in identifying more severe injuries that require medical intervention (Matz 2003). Neuroimaging has also been used to demonstrate that more complicated concussions (i.e., with positive imaging findings) are more similar to moderate TBI than are concussions without imaging findings (Williams et al. 1990). Children with neuroimaging abnormalities following mild TBI have been shown to display more postconcussion disorder symptoms than those without neuroimaging abnormalities (Taylor et al. 2010) and to show poorer neuropsychological outcomes (Levin et al. 2008). More modern neuroimaging procedures that assess brain structure (i.e., diffusion tensor imaging, susceptibility weighted imaging) or function (e.g., functional MRI, magnetic source imaging (MSI), positron emission tomography, and single-photon emission CT) may hold promise in the assessment of concussions and mTBI (Ashwal 2010; Hunt and Asplund 2010; Mendez et al. 2005), but standards for clinical procedures in individual cases have yet to be developed at this time. Several recent studies have provided some support for the use of advanced imaging techniques in predicting neurobehavioral outcomes following mTBI (Levin et al. 2004; Newsome et al. 2008), but this remains experimental.

2.4.2 Grading Systems

Although grading systems were once popular in the sports medicine literature to make return to play decisions, their use has not gained wide acceptance in other clinical settings. First, empirical evidence for the majority of these grading systems is lacking (Anderson et al. 2006). In most medical settings, the criteria used in the grading systems cannot be practically gathered. For example, the AAN grading system requires documenting the duration of concussion symptoms and mental status abnormalities immediately following injury. This can be accomplished on the athletic field where team physicians and athletic trainers are available immediately after the injury and can monitor the athlete's functioning postacutely. In the context of nonsports-related concussions, however, the patient often does not receive immediate medical attention to document acute mental status abnormalities and the exact time of injury is sometimes not available to assist with documenting duration of symptoms. Finally, the majority of concussion grading systems are based on factors such as LOC and PTA, which often cannot be reliably documented in concussion populations.

2.4.3   Concussion Versus Mild TBI

As indicated in the definition section of this chapter, a major controversy exists regarding the distinction, if any, between concussion and mTBI. Is concussion the same as mTBI or do they represent different conditions? Is concussion simply a variant of mTBI? How does concussion fit into the broader TBI spectrum? A comparison of the ACRM and WHO definitions (see Table 2.1) and the TBI severity spectrum (see Table 2.2) suggests that, based on length of PTA, some injuries that ACRM and WHO define as "mild" would be considered "moderate TBI" using traditional severity ratings. This definitional confusion needs to be resolved to advance empirical and clinical understanding of concussions.

2.4.4   Complicated mTBI

Many authors and clinicians have used the term "complicated mTBI" to distinguish mild head injuries (or concussions) that result in positive neuroimaging findings. Research has provided evidence in support of the distinction, finding that individuals with complicated mTBI are more similar to those with moderate TBI in regards to measures of neurobehavioral and neuropsychological outcomes (Levin et al. 2008; Taylor et al. 2010; Williams et al. 1990). An alternative approach would be to label any injury with neuroimaging evidence of parenchymal injury as moderate TBI. This issue needs further empirical attention, especially in pediatric populations.

2.4.5   Young Children with Concussion

The vast majority of research on concussion and mTBI has been conducted with adolescents and young adults. This leaves a major gap in our understanding of the clinical presentation and sequelae of these injuries in young children (Kirkwood et al. 2006). Fortunately several investigators have begun to examine concussions in this population (Mittenberg et al. 1997; Thiessen and Woolridge 2006; Yeates et al. 1999, 2009; Yeates and Taylor 2005). Several controversial issues have emerged in research and clinical endeavors with pediatric concussion. Assessing injury severity in infants and young children can be difficult when relying on traditionally adult measures such as GCS and PTA (Yeates 2010). The GCS relies on verbal and motor components that may not be developmentally appropriate for young children. Attempts have been made to adapt the GCS to younger populations (see Durham et al. 2000). Measuring PTA in young children often relies on report from either parents or medical staff because young children may not be able to reliably provide self-report of memories around the time of injury. Objective measures of PTA have been developed, such as the Children's Orientation and Amnesia Test (COAT, Ewing-Cobbs et al. 1990), although assessing PTA in preschool children is problematic. Specific grading systems have not been developed for pediatric concussion, and it is unclear if pediatric concussions should be classified differently than adolescent and adult concussions.

2.5 Summary

Increased attention has been given to concussions in both research and clinical settings in the past two decades. Despite this increased attention, a consensus has not been reached regarding an exact definition of the term concussion or the classification of concussion severity. Numerous controversies exist with regard to methods of assessing severity of TBI (i.e., LOC, PTA, GCS, etc.) and systems of grading severity within concussion itself (i.e., grading systems). We cannot clearly differentiate a concussion from an mTBI, and it is unclear whether or not an injury can be classified as a concussion if parenchymal injury is present. Most empirical studies have been conducted with adolescents and young adults, leading to a large gap in our knowledge of how to define and classify concussions in infants, preschoolers, and school age children. An emerging body of research is now available about this population; however, more research is needed to guide clinical activities with these groups.

2.6 Key Points

Several definitions exist for concussion, but no consensus has been reached.
There are no specific classification systems for pediatric concussion.
There is no consensus regarding the distinction between concussion and mTBI.
There is an emerging literature regarding pediatric concussion and mTBI, but numerous nosological controversies remain.

References

(1966) Committee on Head Injury Nomenclature of the Congress of neurological surgeons: glossary of head injury, including some definitions of injury to the cervical spine. *Clinical Neurosurgery, 12*, 386–394.

American Academy of Neurology. (1997). Practice parameter: The management of concussion in sports (summary statement). Report of the Quality Standards Subcommittee. *Neurology, 48*(3), 581–585.

American Psychiatric Association. (1994). *Diagnostic and Statistical Manual of Mental Disorders* (4th ed.). Washington, D.C.: American Psychiatric Association.

Anderson, T., Heitger, M., & Macleod, A. D. (2006). Concussion and mild head injury. *Practical Neurology, 6*, 342–357.

Ashwal, S. (2010). Neuroimaging in pediatric traumatic brain injury. In V. A. Anderson & K. O. Yeates (Eds.), *Pediatric traumatic brain injury: new directions in clinical and translational research*. New York: Oxford University Press.

Boake, C., McCauley, S. R., Levin, H. S., Contant, C. F., Song, J. X., Brown, S. A., et al. (2004). Limited agreement between criteria-based diagnoses of Postconcussional syndrome. *The Journal of Neuropsychiatry and Clinical Neurosciences, 16*, 493–499.

Boake, C., McCauley, S. R., Levin, H. S., Pedroza, C., Contant, C. F., Song, J. X., et al. (2005). Diagnostic criteria for Postconcussional syndrome after mild to moderate traumatic brain injury. *The Journal of Neuropsychiatry and Clinical Neurosciences, 17*, 350–356.

Bodin, D., & Yeates, K. O. (2010). Traumatic Brain Injury. In R. J. Shaw & D. DeMaso (Eds.), *Textbook of pediatric psychosomatic medicine.* Washington, DC: American Psychiatric Publishing.

Brown, S. J., Fann, J. R., & Grant, I. (1994). Postconcussional disorder: time to acknowledge a common source of neurobehavioral morbidity. *The Journal of Neuropsychiatry and Clinical Neurosciences, 6*, 15–22.

Cantu, R. C. (2001). Posttraumatic retrograde and anterograde amnesia: Pathophysiology and implications in grading and safe return to play. *Journal of Athletic Training, 36*(3), 244–248.

Cantu, R. C. (2006). An overview of concussion consensus statements since 2000. *Neurosurgical Focus, 21*, 1–5.

Carroll, L. J., Cassidy, J. D., Holm, L., Kraus, J., & Coronado, V. G. (2004). Methodological issues and research recommendations for mild traumatic brain injury: the WHO collaborating centre task force on mild traumatic brain injury. *Journal of Rehabilitation Medicine. Supplement, 43*, 113–125.

Colorado Medical Society. (1991). *Report of the Sports Medicine Committee: Guidelines for the Management of Concussion in Sports (revised).* Denver: Colorado Medical Society.

Committee on Quality Improvement, American Academy of Pediatrics (1999) The management of minor closed head injury in children. *Pediatrics, 104*, 1407–1415.

DeMatteo, C. A., Hanna, S. E., Mahoney, W. J., Hollenber, W. J., Hollenberg, R. D., Scott, L. A., et al. (2010). My child doesn't have a brain injury, he only has a concussion. *Pediatrics, 125*, 327–334.

Durham, S. R., Clancy, R. R., Leuthardt, E., Sun, P., Kamerling, S., Dominguez, T., et al. (2000). CHOP infant coma scale ("Infant Face Scale"): A novel coma scale for children less than two years of age. *Journal of Neurotrauma, 17*, 729–737.

Esselman, P. C., & Uomoto, J. M. (1995). Classification of the spectrum of mild traumatic brain injury. *Brain Injury, 9*, 417–424.

Ewing-Cobbs, L., Levin, H. S., Fletcher, J. M., Miner, M. E., & Eisenberg, H. M. (1990). The children's orientation and amnesia test: relationship to severity of acute had injury and to recovery of memory. *Neurosurgery, 27*, 683–691.

Falk, A. C., Cederfjäll, C., von Wendt, L., & Söderkvist, B. K. (2005). Management and classification of children with head injury. *Child's Nervous System, 21*, 430–436. doi:10.1007/s00381-005-1142-4.

Gordon, K. E., Dooley, J. M., & Wood, E. P. (2006). Descriptive epidemiology of concussion. *Pediatric Neurology, 34*, 376–378.

Hunt, T., & Asplund, C. (2010). Concussion assessment and management. *Clinical Journal of Sports Medicine, 29*, 5–17.

Kirkwood, M. W., Yeates, K. O., & Wilson, P. E. (2006). Pediatric sport-related concussion: a review of the clinical management of an oft-neglected population. *Pediatrics, 117*, 1259–1371.

Langlois, J. A., Rutland-Brown, W., & Thomas, K. E. (2006). *Traumatic Brain injury in the United States: Emergency department visits, hospitalizations, and deaths.* Atlanta, GA: Centers for Disease Control and Prevention, National Center for Injury Prevention and Control.

Levin, H. S., Hanten, G., Roberson, G., Li, X., Ewing-Cobbs, L., Dennis, M., et al. (2008). Prediction of cognitive sequelae based on abnormal computed tomography findings in children following mild traumatic brain injury. *Journal of Neurosurgery. Pediatrics, 1*, 461–470.

Levin, H. S., Zhang, L., Dennis, M., Ewing-Cobbs, L., Schachar, R., & Hunter, J. V. (2004). Psychosocial outcome of TBI in children with unilateral frontal lesions. *Journal of International Neuropsychological Society, 10*, 305–316.

Makdissi, M. (2009). Is the simple versus complex classification of concussion a valid and useful differentiation? *British Journal of Sports Medicine, 43*(Suppl 1), i23–i27. doi: 10.1136/bjsm. 2009.058206.

Matz, P. G. (2003). Classification, diagnosis, and management of mild traumatic brain injury: a major problem presenting in a minor way. *Seminars in Neurosurgery, 14*(2), 125–130.

McCrory, P., Johnston, K., Meeuwisse, W., Aubry, M., Cantu, R., Dvorak, J., et al. (2005). Summary and agreement statement of the 2nd International Conference on Concussion in Sport, Prague 2004. *British Journal of Sports Medicine, 39*, 196–204.

McCrory, P., Meeuwisse, W., Johnston, K., Dvorak, J., Aubry, M., Molloy, M., et al. (2009). Consensus statement on concussion in sport 3rd International Conference on Concussion in Sport Held in Zurich, November 2008. *Clinical Journal of Sports Medicine, 19*, 185–195.

Mendez, C. V., Hurley, R. A., Lassonde, M., Zhang, L., & Taber, K. H. (2005). Mild traumatic brain injury: Neuroimaging of sports-related concussion. *The Journal of Neuropsychiatry and Clinical Neurosciences, 17*, 297–303.

Mild Traumatic Brain Injury Committee, ACoRM., Head Injury Interdisciplinary Special Interest Group. (1993). Definition of mild traumatic brain injury. *The Journal of Head Trauma Rehabilitation, 8*(3), 86–87.

Mittenberg, W., & Strauman, S. (2000). Diagnosis of mild head injury and the Postconcussional syndrome. *The Journal of Head Trauma Rehabilitation, 12*(2), 783–791.

Mittenberg, W., Wittner, M. S., & Miller, L. J. (1997). Postconcussional syndrome occurs in children. *Neuropsychology, 11*, 447–452.

Newsome, M. R., Steinberg, J. L., Scheibel, R. S., Troyanskaya, M., Chu, Z., Hanten, G., et al. (2008). Effects of traumatic brain injury on working memory-related brain activation in adolescents. *Neuropsychology, 22*, 419–425.

Ruff, R. M., & Jurica, P. (1999). In search of a unified definition for mild traumatic brain injury. *Brain Injury, 13*(12), 943–952.

Slobounov, S. (2008). Concussion classification: historical perspective and current trends. In *Injuries in athletics: Causes and consequences* (pp. 399–414). Boston, MA: Springer.

Tator, C. H. (2009). Let's standardize the definition of concussion and get reliable incidence data. *Canadian Journal of Neurological Sciences, 36*, 405–406.

Taylor, H. G., Dietrich, A., Nuss, K., Wright, M., Rusin, J., Bangert, B., et al. (2010). Post-concussive symptoms in children with mild traumatic brain injury. *Neuropsychology, 24*, 148–159.

Teasdale, G., & Jennett, B. (1974). Assessment of coma and impaired consciousness: A practical scale. *Lancet, 2*, 81–84.

Thiessen, M. L., & Woolridge, D. P. (2006). Pediatric minor closed head injury. *Pediatric Clinics of North America, 53*, 1–26. doi:10.1016/j.pcl.2005.09.004.

Willer, B., Dumas, J., Hutson, A., & Leddy, J. (2004). A population based investigation of head injuries and symptoms of concussion of children and adolescents in schools. *Injury Prevention, 10*, 144–148.

Williams, D. H., Levin, H. S., & Eisenberg, H. M. (1990). Mild head injury classification. *Neurosurgery, 27*, 422–428.

World Health Organization. (1992). *The ICD-10 classification of mental and behavioural disorders: diagnostic criteria for research*. Geneva: World Health Organization.

Yeates, K. O. (2010). Traumatic brain injury. In K. O. Yeates, M. D. Ris, H. G. Taylor, & B. F. Pennington (Eds.), *Pediatric neuropsychology: research, theory, and practice* (2nd ed., pp. 112–146). New York: Guilford.

Yeates, K. O., Luria, J., Baertkowski, H., Rusin, J., Martin, L., & Bigler, E. D. (1999). Postconcussive symptoms in children with mild closed head injuries. *The Journal of Head Trauma Rehabilitation, 14*, 337–350.

Yeates, K. O., & Taylor, H. G. (2005). Neurobehavioral outcomes of mild head injury in children and adolescents. *Pediatric Rehabilitation, 8*, 5–16.

Yeates, K. O., Taylor, H. G., Rusin, J., Bangert, B., Dietrich, A., Nuss, K., et al. (2009). Longitudinal trajectories of Postconcussive symptoms in children with mild traumatic brain injuries and their relationship to acute clinical status. *Pediatrics, 123*, 735–743.

Chapter 3
Sports-Related Concussion

Amy E. Valasek and Teri Metcalf McCambridge

3.1 Introduction

A sports-related concussion is defined as a complex pathophysiologic process affecting the brain induced by traumatic biomechanical forces (McCrory et al. 2009). Sports-related concussion has received greater attention in the last decade as research has provided insight into the negative impacts if improperly diagnosed or poorly treated. Ten years ago, 300,000 sports-related traumatic brain injuries with associated loss of consciousness were reported annually in the USA (Centers for Disease Control and Prevention (CDC) 1997). With more knowledge, education, and greater sports participation in youth athletics, the actual annual overall incidence of concussion is estimated to be closer to 1.6–3.6 million annually in the USA (CDC 1997). There is growing evidence that the pediatric athlete (aged 5–18 years) is extremely vulnerable to concussion. Consideration of the pediatric athlete as a different entity from an adult athlete is essential. This chapter reviews the current epidemiology, age relationship, gender relationship, and sport-specific risk related to pediatric sports-related concussion.

A.E. Valasek (✉)
Department of Orthopedics, Pediatric Division, Johns Hopkins Hospital,
White Marsh, MD, USA
e-mail: avalase1@jhmi.edu

T.M. McCambridge
Director of Sports Medicine Division, Cincinnati Children's Hospital Medical Center,
Cincinnati, OH, USA

J.N. Apps and K.D. Walter (eds.), *Pediatric and Adolescent Concussion:*
Diagnosis, Management and Outcomes, DOI 10.1007/978-0-387-89545-1_3,
© Springer Science+Business Media, LLC 2012

3.2   Epidemiology in Pediatric Athletics

Approximately 30–45 million children participate in recreational sport programs annually based on data obtained from National Alliance for Youth Sports and National Council for Youth Sports (Gioia et al. 2009). The CDC reports that 200,000 traumatic brain injuries are seen in the US Emergency Departments yearly and 65% are thought to be children aged 5–18 years (CDC 2007). The exact incidence of pediatric sports-related concussion is unknown, although the CDC estimates about 20% of the 1.5 million head injuries treated annually are sports related (Table 3.1).

Concussion recognition by coaches, parents, and athletes continues to be suboptimal. At the high-school level, it is believed that many concussions are unreported by the athlete for fear of being held from participation or due to lack of recognition, as some children attribute the injury as "just getting my bell rung." Additionally, a recent survey of youth sport coaches revealed that 42% believed that concussion occurs only with loss of consciousness and 25% would allow a symptomatic child return to play (Valovich McLeod et al. 2007). This misunderstanding of concussion demonstrates the difficulty in obtaining true incidence data. It also highlights the importance of education of all coaches and parents at the recreational youth level to recognize signs and symptoms of concussion and understand the consequences of improper return to play.

There are many difficulties in completing epidemiology studies on sports-related concussion. First, athletes may not recognize that they have an injury and may not report their injury to health care providers. Athletes are often treated in many different arenas, from the school athletic trainer to urgent care clinics and emergency departments to their primary care physician to specialty clinics involving neurosciences and sports medicine. However, data continues to show that sports-related concussion injuries are on the rise.

Table 3.1 Estimated annual number of emergency department visits for nonfatal traumatic brain injuries related to sports and recreational activities for ages 5–18 years, by activity

Activity	Number of TBIs	95% Confidence interval
Bicycle	23,405	16,860–29,950
Football	20,293	16,255–24,332
Basketball	11,506	8,528–14,485
Playground	10,414	7,185–13,644
Soccer	7,667	4,747–10,588
Baseball	7,433	5,440–9,426
All-terrain vehicle	5,220	2,462–7,979
Hockey (ice, roller, field, street)	4,111	1,523–6,699
Skateboard	4,408	2,561–6,255
Swimming/diving	3,846	2,325–5,367
Horseback riding	2,648	1,593–3,704

Adapted from CDC (2007)

A recent study evaluated the change in emergency department visits for sport-related concussion from 1997 to 2007 (Bakhos et al. 2010). In 8–13-year olds, the number of visits doubled while in 14–19-year olds the visit numbers increased by over 200%. A new injury surveillance system for high schools, High School Reporting Information Online (HS RIO), has been set up in conjunction with the National Federation of State High School Associations (NFHS) to track injuries in the high-school athlete. The data being collected is helping identify injury rates at the high-school level. During the 2005–2006 school year, it was estimated that concussions represented 8.9% of all injuries (Gessel et al. 2007).

3.3   Age

Evidence has established children's increased vulnerability to the effects of traumatic brain injury. Animal research on rodents has further solidified this theory by repeatedly demonstrating younger rodents' increased susceptibility to brain injury and more prolonged recovery time. A group of concussed high-school athletes recovered more slowly to cognitive baseline than college athletes on neuropsychological testing by approximately 1 week (Field et al. 2003). Furthermore, professional NFL athletes were found to recover within 2–3 days based on neuropsychological tests (Pellman et al. 2006a). The disparity in the normalization of cognitive function is significant for proper concussion management based on age. Multiple studies have since shown that high-school athletes often return to cognitive baseline within 30 days of injury (Collins et al. 2002, 2003; McCrea et al. 2004), whereas college athletes normalize to baseline in 7–10 days (Collins et al. 1999; Echemendia et al. 2001; McCrea et al. 2003) and professional athletes in 3–5 days (Pellman et al. 2004, 2006a, b). More importantly, there is a paucity of research focusing on brain recovery after traumatic injury in athletes aged 5–12 years. Many of the symptom assessment tools are not geared to younger pediatric athletes and do not account for developmental level (Gioia et al. 2009). Future focus on these young athletes is essential, and proper symptom assessment tools and neuropsychological tests must be developed for these younger children at different developmental levels.

3.4   Gender Differences

Female participation in athletics has risen exponentially, and historically concussion research focused on the male athlete. Multiple recent prospective surveillance studies have uncovered a greater risk of concussion to the female than male counterparts in comparable sports. An important review pooled ten prospective surveillance studies, critically reviewed the data, and identified three sports felt to be adequately similar between genders (basketball, soccer, and ice hockey) (Dick 2009). The primary populations included high-school, college, and elite athletes.

The review demonstrated statistically significant higher incidence of concussion in female basketball and soccer athletes. Males demonstrated more concussions from direct contact while females showed more concussions from surface or ball contact (Dick 2009). Evidence from HS RIO has suggested that there may be differences between genders with regard to symptoms. For instance, males regularly reported more amnesia and disorientation/confusion than females with concussion (Frommer et al. 2011).

Research has also demonstrated a potential need for modification of the interpretation of neuropsychological testing based on gender alone. Female high-school and college athletes have higher reaction times and greater symptom scores than male counterparts (Broshek et al. 2005). Furthermore, a cohort study by Colvin et al. concluded that female soccer athletes performed worse on postconcussive neurocognitive testing and reported more postconcussive symptoms than male counterparts (Colvin et al. 2009). Also a recent study of children (mean age 14.1 years) showed that concussed girls had significantly higher symptom scores than boys at initial presentation (Blinman et al. 2009).

This data indicates that gender is an important factor in concussion management. The studies emerging demonstrate that female athletes have an increased risk of concussion and potentially poorer functioning on neuropsychological testing. Future endeavors should focus more specifically on uncovering to what extent the gender discrepancy may be hormonal, biochemical at some other level, cultural, or multifactorial in origin.

3.5   High-Risk Sports

Increases in sports participation, intensity, and competition place any athlete at risk of sports-related concussion; however, those deemed as contact sports are the typical culprits. Many surveillance studies over the last decade have examined frequency patterns in various sports. An earlier study supported by the National Athletic Trainers Association (NATA) pooled data from ten high-school sports (boys' football, wrestling, soccer, basketball, baseball, girls' soccer, basketball, softball, field hockey, volleyball) over a 3-year time period (Powell and Barber-Foss 1999). The majority of sports had a higher concussion rate during competition, though volleyball was the exception. Football had the highest concussion rate overall for male high-school athletes. The linebackers, running backs, and offensive line were at the greatest risk. Wrestling was the second highest in concussion frequency in males, with majority occurring during a takedown maneuver. Soccer demonstrated the highest overall concussion rate in female athletes. In both genders, concussions during soccer most frequently occurred from body-to-body collisions while attempting to head the ball.

Ten years later, another surveillance study investigated the epidemiology of concussion in both high-school and collegiate athletes (Gessel et al. 2007). In the nine high-school sports (boys' football, soccer, basketball, wrestling, and baseball; girls' soccer, volleyball, basketball, and softball) studied over one school year, concussions were typically encountered during competitions, mainly with football and girls' soccer. Concussion rates were highest in competition for all sports, except girls' volleyball and softball. The positions of greatest risk were linebackers and running backs in football, goal keepers in boys' soccer, defenders in girls' soccer, guards in girls' basketball, forwards in boys' basketball, takedown position in wrestling, ball contact during baseball, and collisions in softball. Overall, the study showed a higher concussion rate in collegiate sports than high-school counterparts.

The trends in college athletics were further evaluated by the National Collegiate Athletic Association (NCAA) Injury Surveillance System (ISS) in 2007 (Hootman et al. 2007). Over 15 sports were analyzed in the course of a 16-year sample period. Rates of concussion increased significantly by 7% over the sample period, possibly reflecting greater awareness. Of the sports studied, football, men's and women's ice hockey, and women's soccer had the highest rates of concussion.

Noncontact sports, such as cheerleading (or spirit), have been studied as well. Over the past decade, cheerleading has become more specialized with the addition of gymnastic tumbling runs, partner stunts, pyramids, and basket tosses. The epidemiology was investigated over a 1-year study period from an Internet-based ISS (Shields et al. 2009). Concussions comprised 6% of the stunt-related injuries reported. Collegiate cheerleaders had a higher concussion frequency than the younger cheerleaders, perhaps related to the difficulty of skills and maneuvers performed.

The majority of sports-related injuries in both genders appear to be sustained during game competitions rather than practice. Prevention initiatives must focus on instituting and enforcing rules and policies developed for each sport. One observational cohort study gathered data over two seasons of sports participation for children aged 7–13 years (Radelet et al. 2002). Children participating in community baseball, softball, soccer, and football demonstrated a relatively low concussion injury rate compared to other injury types, such as contusions, lacerations, sprains, and fractures. The concussion incidence in this population likely is lower secondary to underreporting and underidentification. Future studies are warranted to uncover the true epidemiology in the younger athlete.

3.6 Summary

Sports-related concussion has no boundaries related to age, gender, and type of sport, so future work must focus on education of the entire athletic community. It is imperative for health care providers to educate parents, coaches, and youth athletes about concussion signs and symptoms. There still are many misconceptions in the community regarding concussion which place young athletes at risk.

3.7 Key Points

A child with a concussion should be managed differently than an adult athlete.

The younger the age of the child, the more vulnerable the brain is to concussion and the longer the time required to return to cognitive baseline.

Player-to-player contact during competition appears to be responsible for the majority of concussions.

In sports played by both genders, girls demonstrate higher concussion rates than male counterparts at both high-school and collegiate levels.

References

Bakhos, L. L., Lockhart, G. R., et al. (2010). Emergency department visits for concussion in young athletes. *Pediatrics, 126*(3), e550–e556.

Blinman, T. A., Houseknecht, E., Snyder, C., et al. (2009). Postconcussive symptoms in hospitalized pediatric patients after mild tarumatic brain injury. *Journal of Pediatric Surgery, 44*, 1223–1228.

Broshek, D. K., Kaushik, T., Freeman, J. R., et al. (2005). Sex differences in outcome following sports-related concussion. *Journal of Neurosurgery, 102*, 856–863.

Centers for Disease control and Prevention (CDC). (1997). Sports-related recurrent injuries in United States. *MMWR Morbidity and Mortality Weekly Report, 46*, 224–227.

Centers for Disease Control and Prevention (CDC). (2007). Nonfatal traumatic brain injuries from sports and recreation activities – United States 2001–2005. *MMWR Weekly, 56*(29), 733–737.

Collins, M., Field, M., Lovell, M., et al. (2003). Relationship between postconcussion headache and neuropsychological performance in high school athletes. *American Journal of Sports Medicine, 31*, 168–173.

Collins, M. W., Grindel, S., Lovell, M. R., et al. (1999). Relationship between concussion and peuropsychological performance in college football players. *Journal of American Medical Association, 282*, 964–970.

Collins, M. W., Lovell, M. R., Iverson, G. L., et al. (2002). Cumulative effects of concussion in high school athletes. *Neurosurgery, 51*, 1175–1181.

Colvin, A. C., Mullen, J., Lovell, M. R., et al. (2009). The role of concussion history and gender in recovery from soccer related concussion. *American Journal of Sports Medicine, 37*, 1699–1704.

Dick, R. W. (2009). Is there a gender difference in concussion incidence and outcomes? *British Journal of Sports Medicine, 43*(suppl 1), i46–i50.

Echemendia, R., Putukian, M., Mackin, R., et al. (2001). Neuropsychological test performance prior to and following sports-related mild traumatic brain injury. *Clinical Journal of Sports Medicine, 11*, 23–31.

Field, M., Collins, M. W., Lovell, M. R., et al. (2003). Does age play a role in recovery from sports-related concussion? A comparison of high school and collegiate athletes. *Journal of Pediatrics, 142*, 546–553.

Frommer, L. J., Gurka, K. K., et al. (2011). Sex differences in concussion symptoms of high school athletes. *Journal of Athletic Training, 46*(1), 76–84.

Gessel, L. M., Fields, J. D., Collins, C. L., et al. (2007). Concussions among United States high school and collegiate athletes. *Journal of Athletic Training, 42*(4), 495–503.

Gioia, G. A., Schneider, J. C., Vaughan, C. G., et al. (2009). Which symptom assessments and approaches are uniquely appropriate for paediatric concussion? *British Journal of Sports Medicine, 43*(suppl 1), i13–i22.

Hootman, J. M., Dick, R., & Agel, J. (2007). Epidemiology of Collegiate Injuries for 15 sports: summary and recommendations for injury prevention initiatives. *Journal of Athletic Training, 42*(2), 311–319.

McCrea, M., Guskiewicz, K. M., Marshall, S. W., et al. (2003). Acute effects and recovery time following concussion in collegiate football players. *Journal of American Medical Association, 290*, 2556–2563.

McCrea, M., Hammeke, T., et al. (2004). Unreported concussion in high school football players: implications for prevention. *Clinical Journal of Sports Medicine, 14*, 13–17.

McCrory, P., Meeuwisse, W., Johnston, K., et al. (2009). Consensus Statement on concussion in Sport. The 3 rd International Conference on Concussion is sport. *British Journal of Sports Medicine, 43*(suppl 1), 76–90.

Pellman, E. J., Lovell, M. R., Viano, D. C., et al. (2004). Concussion in professional football: neuropsychological testing – part 6. *Neurosurgery, 55*, 1290–1305.

Pellman, E. J., Lovell, M. R., Viano, D. C., et al. (2006a). Concussion in professional football: recovery of NFL and high school athletes assessed by computerized neuropsychological testing – part 12. *Neurosurgery, 58*(2), 263–274.

Pellman, E. J., Lovell, M. R., Viano, D. C., et al. (2006b). MTBI in professional football: recovery in NFL and high school athletes. *Neurosurgery*, 58(2):263–274.

Powell, J. W., & Barber-Foss, K. D. (1999). Traumatic brain injury in high school athletes. *Journal of American Medical Association, 282*(10), 958–963.

Radelet, M. A., Lephart, S. M., et al. (2002). Survey of injury rate for children in community sports. *Journal of Pediatrics, 110*(3), 1–11.

Shields, B. J., Fernandez, S. A., & Smith, G. A. (2009). Epidemiology of cheerleading stunt-related injuries in United States. *Journal of Athletic Training, 44*(6), 586–594.

Valovich McLeod, T. C., Schwartz, C., & Bay, R. C. (2007). Sports-related concussion misunderstanding amoung youth coaches. *Clinical Journal of Sports Medicine, 2007*(17), 140–141.

Chapter 4
Biomechanics and Pathophysiology of Concussion

Michael McCrea and Mathew R. Powell

4.1 Introduction

The basic and clinical science of concussion has advanced more over the last two decades than it had in the prior 50 years, due in large part to major technological advances that enable innovative approaches to studying the biomechanics, neurophysiology, and functional neuroanatomy that underlie the clinical presentation of concussion in humans. An abundance of research over the last 10 years has illustrated a clear neuropathophysiology of concussion, while also clarifying the expected time course for the brain's eventual return to normal physiological functioning after concussion. A more informed perspective into the basic mechanisms of concussion ultimately moves us closer and closer to answering the pressing question: *what is the true natural history of concussion?* Furthermore, these advances in the basic science of concussion also now put us in a much better position to interpret the persistent clinical effects of concussion and inform our understanding of post-concussion syndrome (PCS). This chapter will review the current scientific literature on the biomechanics and pathophysiology of concussion, including special considerations relevant to pediatric concussion.

M. McCrea (✉)
Departments of Neurosurgery and Neurology,
Medical College of Wisconsin, Milwaukee, WI, USA
e-mail: mmccrea@mcw.edu

M.R. Powell
Neuropsychology Department, Minocqua Behavioral Health,
Marshfield Clinic, Minocqua, WI, USA

J.N. Apps and K.D. Walter (eds.), *Pediatric and Adolescent Concussion:
Diagnosis, Management and Outcomes*, DOI 10.1007/978-0-387-89545-1_4,
© Springer Science+Business Media, LLC 2012

4.2 Review of Current Research

4.2.1 Biomechanics of Concussion

Reconstructing the event or accident that is considered the cause of a patient's presenting injuries is a critical component of any injury examination. This exercise is perhaps no more difficult than in the case of concussion, where often there are no eyewitnesses and the patient is unable to provide a credible report due to a period of unconsciousness or posttraumatic amnesia that confounds their account of the incident. As a result, clinicians are often left with the challenge of determining whether or not the accident in question was sufficient to cause underlying brain injury. In a motor vehicle accident scenario, it is common to ascertain where the patient was positioned in the vehicle, whether they were belted, how fast the vehicle was traveling, the crash orientation (e.g., rear-ended vs. broadsided vs. rollover), and the nature of any direct impact to the head in the accident – all in hopes of reconstructing a biomechanical model for that individual case. In other accident scenarios, it is equally important to establish aspects of acceleration and deceleration, translational and rotational dynamics, and a general sense of injury biomechanics. Historically, establishing a *minimal biomechanical threshold* for traumatic brain injury has been one of the most elusive concepts frustrating biomechanists and neuroscience researchers.

The seminal work by Ommaya and Gennarelli (1974) continues as one of the cornerstones of research on the biomechanics and neuropathology of concussion. These researchers presented a hypothesis for cerebral concussion that outlined the principles underlying the distribution of focal and diffuse effects on neural tissues from cerebral concussion, which correlated with the clinical, experimental, and pathological observations on blunt head trauma from that era. The Ommaya and Gennarelli definition of cerebral concussion referenced clinical, pathophysiological, and biomechanical components as a *"graded set of clinical syndromes following head injury wherein increasing severity of disturbance in level and content of consciousness is caused by mechanically-induced strains affecting the brain in a centripetal sequence of disruptive effect on function and structure. The effects of this sequence always begin at the surfaces of the brain in the mild cases and extend inwards to affect the diencephalic–mesencephalic core at the most severe levels of trauma"*.

The hypotheses of Ommaya and Gennarelli (1974) on the biomechanics and pathophysiology of concussion led to three important predictions. *First*, when the level of trauma is severe enough to produce what is described as traumatic unconsciousness, the extent of simultaneous primary injury in the brain is more severe in cortical and subcortical structures than in the rostral brainstem. *Secondly*, because the mesencephalon is the last to be affected by trauma, primary damage to the rostral brainstem will not occur in isolation in the vast majority of head injuries that are associated with acceleration or deceleration trauma. Primary lesions of the rostral brainstem are rarely found at postmortem, and always in association with more diffuse damage to the brain. In the case of lower grades of cerebral concussion where the patient dies from other causes, Ommaya and Gennarelli hypothesized that isolated primary rostral brainstem lesions should not be found. The *third* prediction from their hypothesis was that, although confusion and disturbances of memory can occur without loss of consciousness, the reverse should never be seen. Every case of head injury with a grade IV cerebral concussion according to their classification system (i.e., paralytic coma with confusion, posttraumatic amnesia, retrograde amnesia) is always associated with a period of posttraumatic amnesia, given that the mesencephalon is less vulnerable than the temporal lobes and limbic system.

Ommaya and Gennarelli went on to reiterate that these three predictions would hold only for the commonly found head injury wherein the head is accelerated or decelerated after impact. The authors cited experimental, clinical, and pathological observations to support the validity of their hypothesis and predictions. From experimental animal models of brain injury, it was asserted that a greater number of traumatic lesions occurred in a more diffusely widespread symmetrical manner from rotational, or angular, than translational, or linear, forces. In their most influential animal study, all the animals in a rotational force group exhibited neurologic evidence of experimental cerebral concussion defined as the sudden onset of paralytic coma or traumatic unconsciousness, while none of the translated force group showed this effect. This study documented the bilateral symmetry and greater severity of all lesions except intracerebral hemorrhages in the rotational force group as compared to the minimally asymmetrical lesion distribution in the translational force group (Ommaya and Gennarelli 1974). Clinically, injuries involving rotational forces also seem to be more significant or severe than linear impacts, in general.

Ommaya and Gennarelli also postulated, from clinical observations, that the majority of concussions do not produce paralytic coma or traumatic unconsciousness, which marked a significant departure from consensus thinking on the topic and a pivotal point in the history of our understanding of concussion. Instead, confusion, amnesia, and any *alteration* in mental status were considered the hallmark characteristics of concussion. They cited the patient who was briefly "dazed" or confused, but continued in a well-coordinated sensory motor activity after a sport-related concussion without subsequent recall of the episode (Yarnell and Lynch 1970, 1973; Ommaya et al. 1973).

Most importantly, the early work by Ommaya and Gennarelli underscored the importance of animal models and the later development of mathematical and physical models as the in vivo laboratory for the study of brain injury biomechanics. There has since been a steady progression in the development of experimental models on traumatic brain injury, including paradigms that illustrate the underlying biomechanical principles of concussion.

More recently, this movement has progressed closer and closer toward answering the elusive unknown of establishing a minimal biomechanical threshold for mild traumatic brain injury (concussion). Recent studies (Ucar et al. 2006) have compared various concussion experimental models, and made recommendations regarding specific weight–height-impact parameters that are most appropriate and simplest for simulating the biomechanics of concussion. This critical evaluation of various experimental models concludes that some models result in effects more reflective of severe head injury, while specific parameters show effects more consistent with concussion.

Over the past decade, several studies have used a combination of video analysis and dummy reenactments of impacts from a sports setting as methods of head acceleration measurement. These studies (Newman et al. 1999, 2000; Pellman et al. 2003a, b) investigated concussive impacts that were recorded on film from two or more different angles. They used this videotape to reconstruct the angle of the impact, speed of the impact, and resultant player kinematics, which provided the necessary information to recreate the impact conditions with instrumented Hybrid-III crash dummies in the biomechanical laboratory.

Pellman and colleagues have published a series of reports on concussion in professional football, including data on the location and direction of helmet impacts (Pellman 2003; Pellman et al. 2003a, b). In a 2003 report (Pellman et al. 2003a), 31 impacts were constructed with the helmeted Hybrid-III dummies involving 25 concussions. This study was the first to illustrate the location, direction, and severity of helmet impacts causing concussion in National Football League (NFL) American football players, as defined by analysis from game video and laboratory reconstruction. From these reconstructions, concussion occurred with the lowest peak head acceleration in facemask impacts at 78 g (±18 g) versus an average of 107–117 g for impacts on other quadrants of the head. There was also significantly higher head acceleration for concussed versus nonconcussed players.

In 2004, Zhang et al. (2004) attempted to delineate injury causation and establish a meaningful injury criterion through the use of actual field accident data from mild traumatic brain injuries in American football, providing what the authors referred to as a unique living "laboratory" to study concussion biomechanics and tolerance levels in humans, with possible extrapolation to the general population. Again, accident reconstruction using an anatomically detailed model facilitated the prediction of the extent and severity of brain response as a consequence of a particular impact.

Zhang and colleagues assert that their approach was unlike previous studies which proposed tolerance limits for human head injury based on input kinematics either scaled from animal data or noninjurious volunteer test results. A total of 24 head-to-head field collisions that occurred in professional football games were duplicated, using a validated finite element human head model. Injury predictors and injury levels were analyzed based on resulting brain tissue responses and were correlated with the site and occurrence of concussion. Predictions indicated that the sheer stress around the brainstem region could be an injury predictor for concussion, and statistical analyses were performed to establish a new brain injury tolerance level. Specifically, based on linear logistic regression analyses, the predicted sheer stress response in the upper brainstem was the best injury predictor over the other brain response parameters. A sheer stress of 7.8 kPa was proposed as the tolerance level for a 50% probability of sustaining a concussion. Contrary to earlier studies, their analysis indicated that the translational head acceleration had a greater influence on intracranial pressure response in comparison with rotational acceleration, and the sheer stress in the central part of the brain was more sensitive to rotational acceleration than to translational acceleration.

Zhang et al. concluded that if the head was exposed to a combined translational and rotational acceleration, with impact duration of between 10 and 30 milliseconds

Table 4.1 Probabilities of concussive injury associated with levels of translational and rotational acceleration

Probability of concussion (%)	Translational acceleration (g)	Rotational acceleration (rad/s^2)
25	66	4.6×10^3
50	82	5.9×10^3
80	106	7.9×10^3

Zhang et al. (2004)

(ms), the suggested tolerable reversible brain injury level was less than 85 g for translational acceleration. The maximum resultant translational acceleration at the center of gravity and probabilities of concussion are listed in Table 4.1.

Other researchers (Brolinson et al. 2006) have argued that dependence on video reconstruction and dummy reenactments creates an indirect measure of head acceleration that is limited by dummy biofidelity assumptions and validation from 30 Hz video. In addition, previous research has not given real time information on the direction and magnitude of the impacts football players receive. Therefore, there has been a critical need for real time measurement of head accelerations that can be readily applied to a larger number of individuals at risk of TBI exposure (e.g., athletes participating in collision sports). Recognizing the limitations of video reconstruction and dummy reenactments, more recent technologies have focused on an innovative in-helmet system that measures and records linear head acceleration.

Brolinson et al. (2006) conducted a study using the head impact telemetry (HIT) system, an in-helmet system with six spring-mounted accelerometers and an antenna that transmits data via radio frequency to a sideline receiver and laptop computer system. A total of 11,604 head impacts were recorded from a college football team throughout the 2003 and 2004 football seasons during 22 games and 62 practices from a total of 52 players. The incidence of injury data was limited, but the study presented an extremely large data set of human head impacts that provides valuable insight into the lower limits of head acceleration that cause concussion.

The average linear acceleration in the Brolinson study was 20.1 g (±18.7) in the 11,601 impacts that did not result in concussion, which was considerably lower than the average for noninjured players of 60 g (±24 g) previously reported by Pellman et al. (2003b). The Brolinson study, however, included all head impacts during practices and games compared with the selection of more severe open field impacts reported by Pellman et al. (2003b). The Brolinson data from the current study are more similar to the 29.2 g average head impact acceleration measured by Naunheim et al. for high school players that included all impacts, not just the most severe (Naunheim et al. 2000). The three brain injuries that occurred in instrumented players in the Brolinson study had a peak linear head acceleration of 55.7 g, 136.7 g, and 117.6 g, for an average peak linear head acceleration of 103.3 g.

The work of Brolinson and colleagues perhaps is more influential in shedding light on the frequency and magnitude of impacts from routine participation in collision sports than concussive events per se. A pressing question relates to the potential long-term implications of frequent subconcussive impacts in the range of 20–30 g. In a basic sense, it is intriguing to contemplate the question of *how much* (total cumulative exposure from lifetime participation in collision sports) versus *how many* (total number of concussive injuries) in predicting risk for late life neurological problems.

Guskiewicz et al. extended the work of Brolinson, using the HIT system in the study of concussive and nonconcussive impacts in collegiate football players (Guskiewicz et al. 2005; Mihalik et al. 2005, 2006; Bell et al. 2006; McCaffrey et al. 2006; 2006 Personal communication with K. Guskiewicz). As part of an ongoing study, more than 27,000 impacts were recorded and analyzed for all exposures in games and practice during a single season. This study also allowed analysis of impact frequency and magnitude, while correlating biomechanical instrumentation data with clinical assessment measures following concussion. In total, nine concussions were observed in HIT-equipped players. The average magnitude of concussion impacts was 95 g, with a range of 60–120 g. Six of the nine concussive events had peak accelerations in excess of 95 g. This compares to less than 1% of the 27,000 nonconcussive impacts that had a peak head acceleration in excess of 95 g. It also should be pointed out, however, that even the overwhelming majority of impacts greater than 80 g did not result in concussion, suggesting that a minimum threshold of translational force in this range is necessary but not solely sufficient to cause concussion.

In summary, several studies using video reconstruction, technologically advanced crash dummies, or even live instrumentation of human sports participants now provide us with data that start to establish a minimal threshold of peak head acceleration that provides valuable insight into the lower limits of head acceleration that cause mild traumatic brain injury. Across studies, there is suggestion of a linear g minimum threshold in the range of 80–100 g. The influence of rotational forces, however, must be considered in this equation as a mediating factor that may lower the necessary threshold of a translational force that causes concussion. As suggested years ago by Ommaya and Gennarelli (1974), the addition of rotational forces greatly increase the likelihood of concussion.

In real world terms, it has been suggested that a 100-g translational force is equivalent to a 25-miles per hour motor vehicle collision into a brick wall, striking one's head against the dash. Instrumentation advancements now provide a first-ever laboratory opportunity to study the biomechanics of concussion in vivo, and allow us to correlate biomechanical data with clinical measures of effects and recovery associated with concussion. In a clinical setting, these data suggesting a minimal biomechanical threshold for the occurrence of concussion should be considered when determining if the accident in question was sufficient to cause brain injury and whether the biomechanics correlate with the severity of the patient's clinical presentation.

4.2.2 Special Considerations on the Biomechanics of Concussion in Pediatric Populations

In general, the biomechanical dynamics of concussion are similar across the lifespan, based largely on the common factor that most injuries involve rotational acceleration and/or deceleration forces that stress or strain the brain tissue, vasculature, and other neural matter (Barth et al. 2001; McCrory et al. 2001). Some unique elements, however, should be considered in the pediatric population. First, we know that the structural maturity of both the body and the brain differ between younger (developing) and older (mature) individuals. Therefore, it is commonly held that the specific effects of any applied force will be age-dependent to some extent. In a 2006 report, Kirkwood et al. summarized the literature on the uniqueness of the pediatric brain by describing the developmental factors such as brain water content, cerebral blood volume, level of myelination, skull geometry, and suture elasticity undoubtedly affect the biomechanics of concussive injury, although exactly how remains largely undetermined (Thibault and Margulies 1998; Gefen et al. 2003; Prins and Hovda 2003; Bauer and Fritz 2004; Kirkwood et al. 2006).

Kirkwood and colleagues also point out the developmental properties of the brain may also specifically influence the threshold necessary to produce concussive brain injury (Goldsmith and Plunkett 2004). They cite earlier experimental data suggesting that the smaller size of immature brains could require increased force to produce actual cerebral injury (Ommaya et al. 2002). In paradox, other data suggest that once actual injury has occurred, the immature brain is likely to respond less well overall (Kirkwood et al. 2006). Additionally from a biomechanical perspective, the underdeveloped neck and shoulder musculature of children and adolescents may also increase their risk of concussive injury in certain situations, including sports.

4.3 Pathophysiology of Concussion

Scientific advances have overhauled theories of the pathophysiology underlying all forms of neuronal injury, including concussion. The physiology of concussion has been nicely delineated by several scientific breakthroughs in the past decade and summarized in great detail as part of several recent reviews (Shaw 2002; Giza and Hovda 2004). Historically, it was often assumed that the clinical manifestation of signs and symptoms following concussion was due to destruction or sheering of neuronal axons. In contrast to earlier rhetoric that the underlying neurophysiology of concussion is exclusively "diffuse axonal injury (DAI)," radiological and pathological studies now demonstrate that most of the pathophysiology of concussion renders neurons *dysfunctional* but not destroyed (Iverson 2005).

Iverson and colleagues (Iverson 2005; Iverson et al. 2006) have provided excellent reviews of the neuropathology of concussion. They specifically cite the groundbreaking work of Giza and Hovda, which is eloquently summarized in a 2001 report on the pathophysiology of concussion (Giza and Hovda 2001). Iverson et al. (2006) point out, "*It was once considered that excessive acceleration/deceleration forces caused sheer strains on the brain that resulted in tearing or stretching of neurons at the time of the injury. Further, it was considered that brainstem was the focus of injury. Taken together, these studies have led numerous clinicians and researchers to conclude that acceleration/deceleration injuries result in sheer strains within the cranial vault, and these in turn lead to sheering of neurons and blood vessels occurring principally in the brainstem. Although no one doubts the existence of sheering*

Table 4.2 Neurometabolic cascade following traumatic brain injury

1. Nonspecific depolarization and initiation of action potentials
2. Release of excitatory neurotransmitters (EAA's)
3. Massive efflux of potassium
4. Increased activity of membrane ionic pumps to restore homeostatis
5. Hyperglycolisis to generate more adenosine triphosphate (ATP)
6. Lactate accumulation
7. Calcium influx and sequestration in mitochondria leading to impaired oxidative metabolism
8. Decreased energy (ATP) production
9. Calpain activation and initiation of apoptosis
    (a) Axolemmal disruption and calcium influx
    (b) Neurofilament compaction via phosphorylation or sidearm cleavage
    (c) Microtubule disassembly and accumulation of axonally transported organelles
    (d) Axonal swelling and eventual axotomy

Giza and Hovda (2001)
Note: Model applies to all-severity TBI; see text for application of neurometabolic cascade specific to MTBI

strains as the primary pathophysiological mechanism responsible for damage to axons, the pathophysiology sequence that leads to traumatic injury of the neurons is a 'process, not an event.'" (Gennarelli and Graham 1998; Iverson et al. 2006).

Based on an extensive review of the literature, Iverson and colleagues pointed out that cell death following concussion, which is considered extremely rare, reflects a spectrum of necrosis on a continuum between apoptotic, or naturally occurring, and necrotic, or externally caused premature, mechanisms (Voller et al. 2001). They also assert that cell death is closely related to injury severity, where very mild concussions likely produce virtually no permanent damage to cells resulting in long-term symptoms or problems, whereas severe traumatic brain injuries, especially those involving considerable forces, often produce widespread cellular death and dysfunction with clear functional consequences.

Recent research demonstrates that cellular injury does not specifically involve brainstem structures, contrary to previous theories. As Iverson et al. point out, the continuum of injury, at the cellular level, ranges from complete and rapidly reversible cellular dysfunction (in the mildest form of concussion), to slow but complete recovery (moderate TBI), to slow and incomplete recovery, to cell death (severe TBI) (Iverson et al. 2006). At the former end of the continuum, the pattern of complete and rapid reversal of neuronal dysfunction correlates very closely with the natural clinical history of concussion.

In terms of its pathophysiology, concussion is defined as any transient neurologic dysfunction resulting from a biomechanical force (Giza and Hovda 2001). The clinical manifestation of concussion results from sequential neuronal dysfunction due to ionic shifts, altered metabolism, impaired connectivity, or changes in neurotransmission. Collectively, the underlying pathophysiological processes of concussion have been characterized as a "neurometabolic cascade" (Giza and Hovda 2001). The stepwise stages of this process as proposed by Giza and Hovda are summarized in Table 4.2 and illustrated in Fig. 4.1.

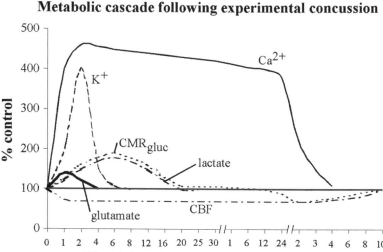

Metabolic cascade following experimental concussion

Fig. 4.1 Neurometabolic cascade following experimental concussion (MTBI)

4.3.1 The "Neurometabolic Cascade"

Upon impact with sufficient biomechanical force to cause concussion (presumably with a minimum threshold of 80–100 g translational acceleration), a process of abrupt and indiscriminant release of neurotransmitters and ionic flux ensues. Excitatory transmitters, including glutamate, bind to the N-methyl-D-aspartate (NMDA) receptor, leading to further neuronal depolarization and efflux of potassium and influx of calcium to affected cells. This process of ionic shift leads to acute and subacute changes in the overall cellular physiology of the brain (Giza and Hovda 2001).

During the acute phase, the sodium potassium pump (Na+, -K+) works exceedingly in an attempt to restore the neuronal membrane to its normal potential. As a result, the sodium potassium pump requires increasing amounts of adenosine triphosphate (ATP), which triggers a dramatic jump in glucose metabolism. In animal studies, increases in glucose metabolism occur almost immediately after fluid percussion injury and persist for up to 30 min in the ipsilateral cortex and hippocampus (Yoshino et al. 1991). The period of increased glucose metabolism is extended perhaps up to several hours and into distant areas of the brain following more severe injury, such as cortical contusion (i.e., "complicated concussion").

This state of hypermetabolism occurs in a state of diminished cerebral blood flow (CBF), with the disparity between glucose supply and demand triggering a generalized cellular energy crisis. CBF is normally tightly coupled to neuronal activity and cerebral glucose metabolism, but may be reduced by 50% in animal fluid percussion models. In a setting of hyperglycolysis, this mismatch in supply and demand results in a potentially damaging energy crisis. This energy crisis is thought to be the likely mechanism for postconcussive vulnerability, making the brain less able to respond adequately to a second injury and potentially leading to long-lasting deficits (Giza and Hovda 2001).

Beyond the initial accelerated glucose utilization, the concussed brain goes into a period of depressed metabolism. Elevated calcium levels persist and can impair mitochondrial oxidative metabolism and amplify the energy crisis. In experimental animal concussion models, the accumulation of calcium is evident within hours and may persist for up to 2–4 days (Cortez et al. 1989; Fineman et al. 1993; McIntosh 1993; Osteen et al. 2001). Persistent and dysregulated calcium accumulation can also contribute to cell death. Intra-axonal calcium flux can disrupt neurofilaments and microtubules that ultimately impair posttraumatic neural connectivity (Giza and Hovda 2001).

The significant influx of calcium can result in myochondrial calcium accumulation and impaired oxidative metabolism, ultimately resulting in energy failure. In animal studies, oxidative metabolism shows a biphasic reduction; in the ipsilateral cortex, a relative reduction on day 1 recovers by day 2, then reoccurs on day 3, and bottoms out on day 5, with recovery by 10 days postinjury. Smaller but more lasting changes have been recorded in the ipsilateral hippocampus, with decreases in oxidative metabolism evident upwards to 10 days postinjury (Hovda et al. 1991).

Cerebral oxidative metabolism normally runs near its maximum in a steady state, so abrupt increase in energy requirements necessitates an increase in glycolysis, or *hyperglycolisis*. Mitochondrial dysfunction associated with impaired oxidative metabolism can lead to reduced ATP production, which provides a second stimulus for increased glycolysis. Increased lactate production in conjunction with decreased lactate metabolism ultimately results in lactate accumulation that can result in neuronal dysfunction by inducing acidosis, membrane damage, altered blood brain barrier permeability, and cerebral edema (Siemkowicz and Hansen 1978; Myers 1979; Kalimo et al. 1981a, b; Gardiner et al. 1982).

Following the initial phase of hyperglycolisis, cerebral glucose use is diminished by 24 h postinjury in animal models and remains below normal levels for 5–7 days in experimental animals (Yoshino et al. 1991). Positron emission tomography (PET) studies in humans show similar decreases in global cerebral glucose metabolism that may last 2–4 weeks post TBI in more severe forms of TBI (Bergsneider et al. 2000), but it is unclear how these effects might present in concussion or milder forms of TBI.

Intracellular magnesium levels are immediately reduced after TBI and remain low for up to 4 days (Vink et al. 1987a, b, 1988; Vink and McIntosh 1990). A decrease in magnesium levels may lead to neuronal dysfunction by multiple pathways; both glycolytic and oxidative generation of ATP are impaired when magnesium levels are low. Also, magnesium is necessary for maintaining the cellular membrane potential and initiating protein synthesis. Finally, low magnesium levels may effectively unblock the NMDA receptor channel more easily, leading to greater influx of calcium and its potential deleterious intracellular consequences.

Giza and Hovda assert that long-term deficits in memory and cognition following all-severity concussion may result from dysfunctional excitatory neurotransmission, including alterations in glutamatergic (NMDA), adrenergic, and cholinergic systems. Specifically, long-term potentiation, an NMDA-dependent measure of neuronal plasticity, may be persistently impaired in the hippocampus after concussion (D'Ambrosio et al. 1998; Sick et al. 1998; Sanders et al. 2000). Concussion may also lead to early changes in choline acetyltransferase activity and degeneration of cholinergic neurons (Schmidt and Grady 1995; Gorman et al. 1996). The biomechanical threshold or magnitude of injury required to trigger this cascade and the specific application to concussion in humans is not entirely clear.

4.3.2 Special Considerations on the Pathophysiology of Concussion in Pediatric Populations

Scientific and clinical evidence suggests that pathophysiological responses after traumatic brain injury are likely age-dependent. For example, the incidence of brain swelling and cerebral edema after moderate and severe brain injury is higher in children than in adults (Aldrich et al. 1992). Recent reviews also suggest that this finding may apply to less severe forms of traumatic brain injury. Specifically, that the pathophysiological dynamics of concussion in young, developing brains may differ from that in adults (Kirkwood et al. 2006).

The most serious consideration to take into account in the pediatric population is the increased risk of rare catastrophic events associated with concussion or mild traumatic brain injury. One of these extremely rare syndromes is often referred to as "second-impact syndrome," a theoretical phenomenon that stems from a case series of catastrophic outcomes associated with concussion, most of which were observed in young athletes. The theoretical model of "second-impact syndrome" is that dysautoregulation of the brain's blood supply is the underlying mechanism, the symptoms of which may include vascular engorgement, diffuse cerebral swelling, increased intracranial pressure, brain herniation, and ultimately coma and death (Cantu 1998). The concept of "second-impact syndrome" remains highly controversial, including debate about whether the second impact actually plays a role in triggering the neurological consequences (McCrory 2001; Cassidy et al. 2004).

Independent of whether these catastrophic cases truly represent "second-impact syndrome," there appears to be general agreement in the scientific community that children are at higher risk of cerebral swelling after even minor head injury and a propensity for structural injury with relatively mild injury, causing some to argue that there may be a different cerebral autoregulatory response to trauma in children and adolescents than in adults (McCrory 2001). There are reports in the literature referring to cases of malignant brain edema syndrome, a rare phenomena observed in athletes in the pediatric age range that consists of a rapid neurologic deterioration from an alert conscious state to coma and sometimes death, minutes to several hours after what appeared to be minor head trauma (Cantu 1998). In pediatric cases, pathology studies show diffuse brain swelling with little or no brain injury; rather than true cerebral edema, a diffuse cerebral swelling appears to be the result of true hyperemia or vascular engorgement.

Although instances of catastrophic outcome after concussion are extremely rare across the lifespan, the increased risk in children and adolescents underscores the value of more conservative injury management strategies in younger populations and the importance of early recognition when any signs of neurologic deterioration are evident after concussion, in hopes of circumventing a neurosurgical emergency or fatal neurologic outcome.

4.4 Influence of Activity on the Pathophysiology of Concussion

Clinicians are often faced with determining a patient's fitness to return to duty, work, or competition after concussion. It is widely accepted in amateur athletics that athletes who sustain a concussion should not return to competition at least until they are symptom-free. When the athlete is asymptomatic, a return to light aerobic exercise is recommended as described in the two agreement statements following the International Concussion in Sport Conferences in Vienna (Aubry et al. 2002) and Prague (McCrory et al. 2005). The protocol, which is based mostly on expert consensus without empirical data, involves an athlete moving through the following exertional steps in 24-h periods (a) light aerobic exercise (e.g., walking or a stationary biking), (b) sport-specific training (e.g., ice skating in hockey or running in soccer), and (3) noncontact training drills (usually heavily exertional). Athletes then progress to contact or full return to play. If the athlete's previously resolved post-concussion symptoms return at any step, the athlete should return to the previous exertion level at which they were last asymptomatic.

It is less clear whether exercising too soon can have short-, medium-, or long-term adverse effects on an injured athlete, warrior, or civilian. Theoretically, if the brain is in a state of neurometabolic crisis and using increased resources to adapt, then exertion (e.g., physical exercise, mental strain, etc.) could worsen the neurometabolic crisis and potentially delay the brain's return to a normal, steady state of cerebral function. Most research designs addressing these issues cannot be implemented with humans, so most of the work in this area has been done with animals.

Griesbach and colleagues have conducted a series of interesting studies relating to exercise following concussion. In one study, 18 rats were injured using a fluid percussion device and then they were returned to cages with or without running wheels (Griesbach et al. 2004a). After a few days, they were sacrificed and molecular markers of plasticity, such as brain-derived neurotrophic factor (BDNF) and Synapsin I were examined. BDNF helps regulate neuronal growth, helps with neuronal survival after injury, and facilitates synaptic function. Synapsin I is involved in synaptic vesicle clustering and release. There was an increase in molecular markers of plasticity measured at 7 days postinjury. However, if injury was followed by acute voluntary exercise, these same molecular markers were decreased.

In this study, early physiological stimulation through voluntary exercise reduced the capacity for plasticity in the injured rat brain.

In a larger study, Griesbach et al. (2004b) administered fluid percussion brain injuries to 161 rats (mean duration of loss of consciousness = 82 s, SD = 54 s; mean duration of apnea = 14 s, SD = 11 s). Some rats were allowed to exercise immediately and some were not given access to a running wheel until 2 weeks postinjury. The rats who were given access to a running wheel immediately did not show positive molecular markers of plasticity and they performed worse on behavioral tasks. The rats who were given access to a running wheel from 14 to 21 days postinjury did show the positive molecular markers and they performed better on the behavioral tasks. Griesbach et al. (2007) utilized a similar methodology but examined both mild and moderate brain injuries. The findings for mild injury were replicated, but moderately injured rats needed to rest longer before they benefited from exercise.

In a recent study, however, Griesbach et al. (2008) obtained results that ran somewhat contrary to their previous work. This study involved a different mechanism of injury (i.e., a cortical contusion injury versus a fluid percussion injury). Molecular improvement *did* occur in injured rats who exercised during the *first week*. However, they did most of their exercising in the last 3 days of that week – they exercised less than the sham rats in the initial days.

Collectively, the series of studies by Griesbach and colleagues suggests that exercise is good for the brain, even the injured brain, but there appears to be an important temporal window. That is, injured rats who exercise too soon do have suppressed molecular markers of plasticity. These studies provide basic science support for the clinical recommendation of complete rest following injury. However, these studies cannot translate directly into clinical recommendations. It is essential to appreciate that the rats first underwent neurosurgery to expose their brain, they were then rendered unconscious (and they typically stopped breathing), and upon regaining consciousness they underwent another neurosurgical procedure prior to being returned to their cages. Uninjured rats went through the same surgical procedures to control for these effects, but the point is that it is extremely difficult to use an animal model to closely approximate a mild concussion experienced in sports or in combat.

Unfortunately, due to obvious methodological and ethical issues and challenges, there is very little research on this topic with humans. Majerske et al. (2008) studied 95 student athletes who were retrospectively assigned into one of the following five groups based on their postconcussion activity level (1) no school or exercise activity (n = 35), (2) school activity only (n = 77), (3) school activity and light activity at home (e.g., slow jogging, mowing the lawn; n = 57), (4) school activity and sports practice (n = 26), (5) school activity and participation in a sports game (n = 9). The group that seemed to function the best cognitively was #3 (school and light activity at home) and the group that functioned the worst cognitively was #5 (school and return to competition). This quasi-experimental retrospective cohort study is interesting and provocative, but does not allow causal inferences. It suggests a relation, however, between activity level and cognitive functioning acutely and postacutely following injury.

4.4.1 Special Considerations on Return to Activity After Concussion in Pediatric Populations

Although we have little in the way of scientific evidence advising us on the true risks incurred by children and adolescents returning to sports or other activities after concussion, the evidence outlined above on the unique dynamics of the developing brain nonetheless move us in the direction of exercising greater caution in our injury management strategies in a younger population.

In a sports setting, the approach to determining a young athlete's fitness to return to competition after concussion is likely similar to that applied with adult athletes, albeit perhaps along a slightly more conservative timeline. The Concussion in Sport Group (CISG) recently issued a recommendation from their expert panel meeting in Zürich Switzerland that youth and adolescent athletes should not resume participation in sport on the same day of their concussion (McCrory et al. 2009). This reasonable and cautious recommendation veers from previous practice. Other sport governing bodies at the high school, collegiate, and professional levels have since adopted this recommendation.

Regardless of age, an accepted standard in the sport medicine community is that no athlete should return to competition until they are completely symptom-free after concussion, under conditions of both rest and maximum exertion. The most common approach is for athletes to progress through a graduated program of exertion over a period of several days after they become symptom-free, during which they demonstrate no recurrence or worsening of symptoms under exertion. Once this is accomplished, the athlete then gradually returns to their sport-specific activities before resuming full participation.

Outside of sports, a similar model should be applied to returning young individuals back to their normal activities at school and otherwise after concussion. Clearly, withholding young children and adolescents from school for extended periods of time is not supported by the literature and may perhaps even create iatrogenic effects that contribute to persistent symptoms, functional deficits, and PCS. The recommended approach is similar to sports in that young individuals should gradually return to their academic, social, and other activities over a period of days, as tolerated without worsening or recurrent symptoms.

The concept of mental or cognitive exertion associated with academic work can follow a similar line to that described above with regard to physical exertion and sports. Again, this transition back to full activity can likely be accomplished within a period of several days in the overwhelming majority of cases. When this transition does not progress as expected, the clinician should give consideration to other noninjury-related factors (e.g., psychological, motivational, etc.) contributing to the protracted course of symptoms or functional difficulties (McCrea et al. 2009).

4.5 Advances in Identifying Biological Mechanisms of Concussion

4.5.1 Serum Biomarkers of Concussion

Along with advances in our understanding of the pathophysiology underlying concussion, there is also pursuit toward identifying biochemical markers that may result in a more sensitive and objective detection of concussion. Several studies have investigated the diagnostic and prognostic value of various biochemical markers, the most common of which are S-100 proteins, neuron-specific enolase (NSE), and cleaved Tau protein (CTP). The most extensive body of research has focused on the S-100B neuroprotein, which is considered a generally reliable marker for brain damage (Ingebrigtsen and Romner 1996, 2002, 2003; Biberthaler et al. 2000; de Kruijk et al. 2001; Herrmann et al. 2001; Mussack et al. 2002a, b).

S-100B is a calcium binding protein which is found in high concentrations in astroglial and Schwann cells, most heavily distributed in the central nervous system (CNS). It is hypothesized that S-100B is rapidly released into cerebrospinal fluid (CSF), and then crosses the blood–CSF barrier upon cell damage. Several studies have reported higher concentrations of S-100B in concussion patients than in non-injured controls (Biberthaler et al. 2001a, b; de Kruijk et al. 2001; Mussack et al. 2002a, b).

Several individual studies have rendered informative findings on the utility of S100B as a marker for concussion. Bazarian et al. (2006) studied the relationship of serum S-100B and C-Tau levels to long-term outcome after mild traumatic brain injury. A total of 35 concussion subjects presenting to the hospital emergency department were studied, with 6-h serum S-100B and C-Tau levels compared to 3-month outcome on postconcussive syndrome questionnaires. A weak correlation was demonstrated between marker levels, and scores on the Rivermead postconcussion questionnaire (S-100B: $R = 0.071$, C-Tau: $R = 0.21$), and there was no statistically significant correlation between acute marker levels and 3-month postconcussive syndrome. Overall, the sensitivity of these two biochemical markers ranged from 43.8 to 56.3%, and the specificity ranged from 35.7 to 71.4%. Bazarian and colleagues concluded that initial serum S-100B and C-Tau levels appear to be poor predictors of 3-month outcome after concussion.

Another concern about the S-100B biochemical marker is its extracranial release, as elevated S-100B levels have been found in nonhead injured patients and healthy sports participants. Bazarian and colleagues (Bazarian et al. 2006) later studied the impact of a correction factor for extracranial release of S-100B based on concomitant creatine kinase (CK) levels. Both CK and S-100B levels were measured in a cohort of 96 concussion patients, which yielded a comparison of corrected S-100B and uncorrected S-100B levels for the prediction of initial head CT, 3-month headache, and 3-month postconcussive syndrome. Corrected S-100B resulted in a statistically significant improvement in the prediction of 3-month headache, but not PCS or initial head CT. Applying a cutoff score that maximized sensitivity improved corrected S-100B's prediction of initial head CT. The researchers concluded that S-100B is poorly predictive of outcome, but that a correction factor using CK may be a valid means of accounting for extracranial release. They also proposed that by increasing the portion of concussion patients correctly categorized as low-risk for abnormal CT, CK-corrected S-100B can further correct the number of unnecessary brain CT scans performed after concussion.

Begaz et al. (2006) recently published a collective review of prospective cohort studies that assess the ability of serum biochemical markers to predict concussion and postconcussive syndrome (PCS). A total of 11 studies assessing S-100B protein, NSE, and CTP were reviewed. The authors concluded that none of these biomarkers consistently demonstrated the ability to predict postconcussive syndrome after concussion, but that a combination of clinical factors in conjunction with biochemical markers may be necessary to develop a comprehensive decision rule that more accurately predicts PCS after concussion.

Iverson et al. (2006) also provided a detailed summary of sensitivity, specificity, and predictive power values of S-100B levels to predict outcome following concussion. A series of studies between 1999 and 2004 was reviewed, with sensitivity values ranging from 80 to 100% and specificity values ranging from 40.5 to 81%. Positive predictive power values ranged from 13 to 40.5, with negative predictive power values between 95.1 and 100. Iverson concluded that the existing body of research suggests that although S-100B is not useful for identifying individuals who are "at risk" of poor outcome from TBI (i.e., positive predictive power), it is useful for identifying those individuals who are "not at risk" of poor outcome from TBI (i.e., negative predictive power; individuals who will have good outcome postinjury).

As a diagnostic tool, the practical implication of this finding from Iverson's review of the literature is that S-100B measures will misidentify a significant portion of individuals "not at risk" (i.e., expected good outcome) as being "at risk," (i.e., potential risk for poor outcome). That is, the test will be positive and they will falsely be labeled as being at risk for poor outcome. Theoretically, this could lead to unnecessary treatment or unnecessary worry for the patient.

In summary, basic science advances have clarified the components and sequence of the pathophysiology underlying the clinical presentation of concussion. Existing evidence suggests a period of metabolic dysfunction that ensues after concussion, with rapid reversal and return to normal brain metabolic function within several days of injury in most cases of concussion, and perhaps extended a bit further in more severe or "complicated" forms of concussion characterized by structural damage visualized on neuroimaging.

This time course is strikingly similar to that illustrated by emerging data plotting the true natural history of the clinical effects of concussion on symptoms, cognition, and general function. Modern technologies also now open the door for the future development of innovative laboratory tests that may provide more objective markers of traumatic brain injury, perhaps with a threshold sufficient for detection of concussion. Further study is required to determine the incremental diagnostic and prognostic utility of biological markers of concussion.

4.5.2 Functional Neuroimaging Studies of Concussion

While other sections will provide a more detailed summary of the literature on neuroimaging techniques in the study of concussion, we will also provide a brief overview here in the context of our understanding surrounding the pathophysiology of these injuries.

Animal studies have described the complex neuropathological processes that come into play following even mild CNS trauma (Raghupathi 2004; Farkas and Povlishock 2007). There have also been several reports of neuropathological findings shortly after concussion in humans who died of other causes (Oppenheimer 1968; Blumbergs et al. 1994, 1995; Goodman and Mattson 1994; Bigler 2004). Neuroimaging, however, has been the mainstay of attempts to understand the neuropathophysiology of human concussion. A full discussion of these efforts is beyond the scope of this paper but has been detailed in recent reviews (Levine et al. 2006; Belanger et al. 2007). Of particular interest are techniques which shed light on two groups (a) individuals studied shortly after injury who have normal conventional structural imaging (such as CT scan or structural MRI), and (b) individuals who do not show the typical recovery pattern.

Two MRI-based techniques show particular promise: diffusion tensor imaging (DTI) and magnetization transfer imaging. DTI is of particular interest in that it is sensitive to subtle changes in white matter integrity. Of particular interest is that fractional anisotropy (FA) values have been shown to correlate with cognitive performance (memory, attention, reaction time) in both healthy controls and individuals with a history of concussion (Niogi et al. 2008a, b).

Arfanakis et al. (2002) reported that five individuals studied within 24 h of a concussion showed reduced fractional anisotropy (FA – a measure of white matter integrity) that was most commonly seen in the corpus callosum and internal capsule. Follow-up scans 1 month later in two of the individuals showed improvement but not complete normalization of the FA values. Inglese et al. (2005) studied 46 patients with concussion (20 of whom within 5 days of injury) and 29 healthy controls. Both concussion groups showed reduced FA and increased mean diffusivity in the corpus callosum, the internal capsule, and the centrum semiovale.

Kraus et al. (2007) performed DTI in 37 individuals with a history of TBI of different severities, 20 of whom had concussion by American Congress of Rehabilitation Medicine criteria (Kay et al. 1993). Compared to 18 healthy controls, the concussion group showed reduced FA in three of 13 regions of interest including the cortico-spinal tract, sagittal striatum, and superior longitudinal fasciculus. Of note is that the concussion group was studied a mean of 92.5 months after injury and had a mean loss of consciousness of about 6 min. Still, the methodology of this study makes it unclear whether a portion of these findings could be accounted for by selection bias (e.g., skewed toward the more severe end of the concussion continuum based on mean LOC), structural brain lesions that occurred at the time of injury (e.g., "complicated" concussion) or nonspecific factors also sensitive to detection by advanced functional imaging techniques. In brief, DTI shows promise as a sensitive and powerful neuroinvestigative tool to advance our understanding of concussion pathophysiology, but further study is required to fully demonstrate its clinical utility in distinguishing the unique (i.e., specific) effects of concussion from other nonspecific changes in brain function.

Bagley et al. (2000) and McGowan et al. (2000) have used magnetization transfer imaging to show regional brain abnormalities following concussion in regions consistent with known neuropathological vulnerability (corpus callosum). In both studies, those individuals with persistent cognitive complaints had demonstrable abnormalities on imaging. In the Bagley study the patients were studied within 1 month of injury. In the McGowan study they were studied within "months" of their injuries and had persistent cognitive complaints.

Functional MRI (fMRI) has been used to study neural mechanisms of cognitive function after concussion. In a fMRI study of 15 concussed high school football athletes within 18 h of injury, Hammeke et al. (2004) found decreased activation in the supplementary motor (SMA) and pre-SMA during a memory scanning paradigm when compared to a matched group of uninjured athletes. The decreased activation occurred largely in players who had a loss of consciousness from their injury and was related to a generalized slowing of selective reaction time. When studied 45 days following injury, the task activation pattern in the concussed players had normalized.

McAllister et al. (1999, 2001, 2006) have suggested that 1 month after concussion, patients show a mismatch of activation and allocation of working memory processing resources, despite cognitive performance that is equivalent to that of healthy controls. Chen et al. (2004) also reported abnormal cerebral activation patterns in 16 concussed athletes studied 1–14 months after injury. Fifteen of the athletes were symptomatic at the time of study. Although performance on the task did not differ from controls, the concussed group showed reduced activation in frontal cortex and increased areas of activation in parietal and temporal regions relative to the controls. This group (Chen et al. 2008) subsequently reported on nine concussed athletes with persistent postconcussive complaints studied on two occasions; 1–9 months after injury and again 9–23 months after the first study. Compared to healthy controls ($n = 6$), the concussed group initially showed reduced dorsolateral prefrontal cortical (DLPFC) activation associated with a working memory task. When reassessed, those concussed athletes whose symptoms had largely resolved ($n = 4$) showed some increased left DLPFC activation relative to the unimproved group. Jantzen et al. (2004) found increased activation associated with cognitive tasks in four concussed athletes (compared to baseline studies and nonconcussed teammates) within a week of injury. Cognitive performance was equivalent between the two groups. More recently, Lovell et al. (2007) also found increased medial frontal and temporoparietal activation associated with a working memory task in 28 concussed student athletes studied about 1 week after injury. Furthermore the degree of activation in this region correlated with length of time to return to play.

In summary, inferences from the above studies must be considered tentative at best in that there are no large scale longitudinal studies of individuals with concussion using the most sensitive available neuroimaging techniques. Variable methods across studies also limit the ability to determine to what extent neuroimaging findings may be influenced by preinjury differences or comorbidities. Nevertheless, neuroimaging research has provided clarity around a number of important elements vital to our understanding of the time course of pathophysiological changes following concussion in humans. The first is that with each advance in imaging technology comes an increase in the sensitivity to detect abnormalities in brain structure and function in the first days to several weeks after concussion. For example conventional MRI demonstrates more lesions than CT scan (Bigler 2005), and more recent MRI-based techniques are more sensitive than the initial T1 and T2 weighted images. Second, within the first month after injury, functional imaging, particularly PET and fMRI show changes in task-associated brain activation even in the absence of abnormal structural imaging. Studies with longer intervals between injury and assessment are more variable. Nevertheless, the recent DTI studies showing increased regions of white matter abnormalities relative to noninjured controls, and correlation of performance with these white matter abnormalities in regions that are biologically plausible, suggest that some longer lasting effects of concussion may be seen in some individuals.

Still, although interpretation of the relationship between persisting symptoms and markers of brain abnormalities noted above seems straightforward when the brain abnormalities are structural in nature (e.g., FA from DTI), more caution is needed when the brain abnormalities are derived from functional imaging techniques because the persisting symptoms may perturb the imaging signal in indirect ways (e.g., be a source of attentional distraction during the imaging study). It is also important to point out that although performance after concussion may return to "normal," the effort required to achieve that performance may be greater than expected, giving rise to a sense of reduced cognitive capacity, and, theoretically, reduced cognitive reserve. Larger longitudinal studies are required to examine these impressions. Additional research is also needed to better understand the natural evolution of brain-related functional adaptation and compensatory mechanisms over time following injury, and to determine why some individuals have persisting brain abnormalities and others do not.

4.6 Summary of Research Findings

In summary, advances in the clinical and basic science of concussion have informed our understanding of the pathophysiology in this century more in the last two decades than ever before. Earlier findings from animal studies and more recent innovative research technologies applied in human studies have significantly increased our understanding of the minimum biomechanical threshold to cause concussion, as well as the complexity and time course of alterations in brain physiology associated with concussion. At present, our pursuit of the quote "perfect biomarker" for concussion remains elusive, but ongoing technological advances are certain to move us closer to this discovery.

4.7 Key Points

Scientific advances over the past decade have filled a previously significant void in our direct knowledge of the biomechanics, neurophysiology, and functional neuroanatomy of concussion, which provides a sound and necessary empirical base on which to build our understanding of the true natural history of clinical effects and recovery after concussion.

Several studies using innovative methods have begun to establish a minimal biomechanical threshold sufficient to cause concussion, which is estimated to be in the range of 80–100 g for translational acceleration; the influence of rotational forces must be considered as a mediating factor that may lower the threshold of pure translational force necessary to cause concussion.

In a clinical setting, evidence of a minimal biomechanical threshold for concussion should be considered when determining if the accident in question was sufficient to cause brain injury and whether the biomechanics correlate with the patient's presenting complaints. The biomechanical dynamics of concussion are common across the lifespan, but several factors should be considered in interpreting the biomechanics of concussive injury in younger populations.

Ground-breaking research has now delineated a rather clear pathophysiology of concussion referred to as the "neurometabolic cascade" and characterized by a stepwise process of ionic shifts, altered brain metabolism, impaired neuronal connectivity, and disruption of normal neurotransmission.

The time course of return to normal cerebral function after the metabolic cascade induced by concussion is not entirely clear, but the bulk of evidence suggests a gradual reversal of physiological abnormalities and return to normal brain metabolic function within days to weeks after concussion.

Young, developing brains appear at heightened risks of extremely rare serious or catastrophic neurological outcomes after concussion, including severe or malignant cerebral swelling and edema. The concept of "second-impact syndrome" remains unclear, including debate over whether catastrophic injury is inherently linked to a second impact.

The evidence-based time course of physiological and metabolic recovery after concussion is strikingly similar to emerging data plotting the true natural history of clinical effects and recovery after concussion (as reviewed in Part 3).

Emerging neuroimaging technologies may further advance our scientific understanding of concussion, but additional research is required to determine the clinical utility, specificity, incremental validity, and prognostic value of these imaging techniques in measuring recovery and predicting outcome after concussion.

References

Aldrich, E. F., Eisenberg, H. M., et al. (1992). Diffuse brain swelling in severely head-injured children. A report from the NIH Traumatic Coma Data Bank. *Journal of Neurosurgery, 76*(3), 450–454.

Arfanakis, K., Haughton, V. M., et al. (2002). Diffusion tensor MR imaging in diffuse axonal injury. *American Journal of Neuroradiology, 23*(5), 794–802.

Aubry, M., Cantu, R., et al. (2002). Summary and agreement statement of the 1st International Symposium on Concussion in Sport Vienna 2001. *Clinical Journal of Sport Medicine, 12*(1), 6–11.

Bagley, L. J., McGowan, J. C., et al. (2000). Magnetization transfer imaging of traumatic brain injury. *Journal of Magnetic Resonance Imaging, 11*(1), 1–8.

Barth, J. T., Freeman, J. R., et al. (2001). Acceleration-deceleration sport-related concussion: the gravity of it all. *Journal of Athletic Training, 36*(3), 253–256.

Bauer, R., & Fritz, H. (2004). Pathophysiology of traumatic injury in the developing brain: an introduction and short update. *Experimental and Toxicologic Pathology, 56*(1–2), 65–73.

Bazarian, J. J., Blyth, B., et al. (2006). Bench to bedside: evidence for brain injury after concussion-looking beyond the computed tomography scan. *Academic Emergency Medicine, 13*(2), 199–214.

Begaz, T., Kyriacou, D. N., et al. (2006). Serum biochemical markers for post-concussion syndrome in patients with mild traumatic brain injury. *Journal of Neurotrauma, 23*(8), 1201–1210.

Belanger, H. G., Vanderploeg, R. D., et al. (2007). Recent neuroimaging techniques in mild traumatic brain injury. *The Journal of Neuropsychiatry and Clinical Neurosciences, 19*(1), 5–20.

Bell, D. R., Mihalik, J. P., et al. (2006). An analysis of head impacts sustained during a complete season by Division I collegiate football players. *Journal of Athletic Training, 41*(2), S40.

Bergsneider, M., Hovda, D. A., et al. (2000). Dissociation of cerebral glucose metabolism and level of consciousness during the period of metabolic depression following human traumatic brain injury. *Journal of Neurotrauma, 17*(5), 389–401.

Biberthaler, P., Mussack, T., et al. (2000). Influence of alcohol exposure on S-100b serum levels. *Acta Neurochirurgica. Supplementum, 76*, 177–179.

Biberthaler, P., Mussack, T., et al. (2001a). Elevated serum levels of S-100B reflect the extent of brain injury in alcohol intoxicated patients after mild head trauma. *Shock, 16*(2), 97–101.

Biberthaler, P., Mussack, T., et al. (2001b). Evaluation of S-100b as a specific marker for neuronal damage due to minor head trauma. *World Journal of Surgery, 25*(1), 93–97.

Bigler, E. D. (2004). Neuropsychological results and neuropathological findings at autopsy in a case of mild traumatic brain injury. *Journal of the International Neuropsychological Society, 10*(5), 794–806.

Bigler, E. D. (2005). Structural neuroimaging in traumatic brain injury. In J. M. M. T. Sliver & S. C. Yudofsky (Eds.), *Textbook of traumatic brain injury*. Washington, DC: American Psychiatric Press.

Blumbergs, P. C., Scott, G., et al. (1994). Staining of amyloid precursor protein to study axonal damage in mild head injury. *The Lancet, 344*(8929), 1055–1056.

Blumbergs, P. C., Scott, G., et al. (1995). Topography of axonal injury as defined by amyloid precursor protein and the sector scoring method in mild and severe closed head injury. *Journal of Neurotrauma, 12*(4), 565–572.

Brolinson, P. G., Manoogian, S., et al. (2006). Analysis of linear head accelerations from collegiate football impacts. *Current Sports Medicine Reports, 5*(1), 23–28.

Cantu, R. C. (1998). Second-impact syndrome. *Clinics in Sports Medicine, 17*(1), 37–44.

Cassidy, J. D., Carroll, L. J., et al. (2004). Incidence, risk factors and prevention of mild traumatic brain injury: results of the WHO Collaborating Centre Task Force on Mild Traumatic Brain Injury. *Journal of Rehabilitation Medicine, 43*(suppl), 28–60.

Chen, J. K., Johnston, K. M., et al. (2004). Functional abnormalities in symptomatic concussed athletes: an fMRI study. *NeuroImage, 22*(1), 68–82.

Chen, J. K., Johnston, K. M., et al. (2008). Recovery from mild head injury in sports: evidence from serial functional magnetic resonance imaging studies in male athletes. *Clinical Journal of Sport Medicine, 18*(3), 241–247.

Cortez, S. C., McIntosh, T. K., et al. (1989). Experimental fluid percussion brain injury: vascular disruption and neuronal and glial alterations. *Brain Research, 482*(2), 271–282.

D'Ambrosio, R., Maris, D. O., et al. (1998). Selective loss of hippocampal long-term potentiation, but not depression, following fluid percussion injury. *Brain Research, 786*(1–2), 64–79.

de Kruijk, J. R., Leffers, P., et al. (2001). S-100B and neuron-specific enolase in serum of mild traumatic brain injury patients. A comparison with health controls. *Acta Neurologica Scandinavica, 103*(3), 175–179.

Farkas, O., & Povlishock, J. T. (2007). Cellular and subcellular change evoked by diffuse traumatic brain injury: a complex web of change extending far beyond focal damage. *Progress in Brain Research, 161*, 43–59.

Fineman, I., Hovda, D. A., et al. (1993). Concussive brain injury is associated with a prolonged accumulation of calcium: a 45Ca autoradiographic study. *Brain Research, 624*(1–2), 94–102.

Gardiner, M., Smith, M. L., et al. (1982). Influence of blood glucose concentration on brain lactate accumulation during severe hypoxia and subsequent recovery of brain energy metabolism. *Journal of Cerebral Blood Flow and Metabolism, 2*(4), 429–438.

Gefen, A., Gefen, N., et al. (2003). Age-dependent changes in material properties of the brain and braincase of the rat. *Journal of Neurotrauma, 20*(11), 1163–1177.

Gennarelli, T. A., & Graham, D. I. (1998). Neuropathology of the head injuries. *Seminars in Clinical Neuropsychiatry, 3*(3), 160–175.

Giza, C. C., & Hovda, D. A. (2001). The neurometabolic cascade of concussion. *Journal of Athletic Training, 36*(3), 228–235.

Giza, C. C., & Hovda, D. A. (2004). The pathophysiology of traumatic brain injury. In M. W. Collins (Ed.), *Traumatic brain injury in sports* (pp. 45–70). Lisse: Swets & Zeitlinger.

Goldsmith, W., & Plunkett, J. (2004). A biomechanical analysis of the causes of traumatic brain injury in infants and children. *The American Journal of Forensic Medicine and Pathology, 25*(2), 89–100.

Goodman, Y., & Mattson, M. P. (1994). Staurosporine and K-252 compounds protect hippocampal neurons against amyloid beta-peptide toxicity and oxidative injury. *Brain Research, 650*(1), 170–174.

Gorman, L. K., Fu, K., et al. (1996). Effects of traumatic brain injury on the cholinergic system in the rat. *Journal of Neurotrauma, 13*(8), 457–463.

Griesbach, G. S., Gomez-Pinilla, F., et al. (2004a). The upregulation of plasticity-related proteins following TBI is disrupted with acute voluntary exercise. *Brain Research, 1016*(2), 154–162.

Griesbach, G. S., Gomez-Pinilla, F., et al. (2007). Time window for voluntary exercise-induced increases in hippocampal neuroplasticity molecules after traumatic brain injury is severity dependent. *Journal of Neurotrauma, 24*(7), 1161–1171.

Griesbach, G. S., Hovda, D. A., et al. (2004b). Voluntary exercise following traumatic brain injury: brain-derived neurotrophic factor upregulation and recovery of function. *Neuroscience, 125*(1), 129–139.

Griesbach, G. S., Hovda, D. A., et al. (2008). Voluntary exercise or amphetamine treatment, but not the combination, increases hippocampal brain-derived neurotrophic factor and synapsin I following cortical contusion injury in rats. *Neuroscience, 154*(2), 530–540.

Guskiewicz, K., Mihalik, J. P., et al. (2005). Recurrent concussion in a collegiate football player equipped with the Head Impact Telemetry System. *Journal of Athletic Training, 40*(2), S81.

Hammeke, T., McCrea, M., et al. (2004). Functional magnetic resonance imaging after acute sports concussion. *Journal of the International Neuropsychological Society, 18*, 168.

Herrmann, M., Curio, N., et al. (2001). Release of biochemical markers of damage to neuronal and glial brain tissue is associated with short and long term neuropsychological outcome after traumatic brain injury. *Journal of Neurology, Neurosurgery, and Psychiatry, 70*(1), 95–100.

Hovda, D. A., Yoshino, A., et al. (1991). Diffuse prolonged depression of cerebral oxidative metabolism following concussive brain injury in the rat: a cytochrome oxidase histochemistry study. *Brain Research, 567*(1), 1–10.

Ingebrigtsen, T., & Romner, B. (1996). Serial S-100 protein serum measurements related to early magnetic resonance imaging after minor head injury. Case report. *Journal of Neurosurgery, 85*(5), 945–948.

Ingebrigtsen, T., & Romner, B. (2002). Biochemical serum markers of traumatic brain injury. *The Journal of Trauma, 52*(4), 798–808.

Ingebrigtsen, T., & Romner, B. (2003). Biochemical serum markers for brain damage: a short review with emphasis on clinical utility in mild head injury. *Restorative Neurology and Neuroscience, 21*(3–4), 171–176.

Inglese, M., Benedetti, B., et al. (2005). The relation between MRI measures of inflammation and neurodegeneration in multiple sclerosis. *Journal of Neurological Sciences, 233*(1–2), 15–19.

Iverson, G. L. (2005). Outcome from mild traumatic brain injury. *Current Opinion in Psychiatry, 18*(3), 301–317.

Iverson, G. L., Lange, R. T., et al. (2006). Mild TBI. In R. D. Zafonte (Ed.), *Brain injury medicine: principles and practice* (pp. 333–371). New York: Demos Medical.

Jantzen, K. J., Anderson, B., et al. (2004). A prospective functional MR imaging study of mild traumatic brain injury in college football players. *American Journal of Neuroradiology, 25*(5), 738–745.

Kalimo, H., Rehncrona, S., et al. (1981a). The role of lactic acidosis in the ischemic nerve cell injury. *Acta Neuropathologica Supplementum, 7*, 20–22.

Kalimo, H., Rehncrona, S., et al. (1981b). Brain lactic acidosis and ischemic cell damage: 2 Histopathology. *Journal of Cerebral Blood Flow and Metabolism, 1*(3), 313–327.

Kay, T., Harrington, D. E., et al. (1993). Definition of mild traumatic brain injury: Report from the Mild Traumatic Brain Injury Committee of the Head Injury Interdisciplinary Special Interest Group of the American Congress of Rehabilitation Medicine. *The Journal of Head Trauma Rehabilitation, 8*(3), 86–87.

Kirkwood, M. W., Yeates, K. O., et al. (2006). Pediatric sport-related concussion: a review of the clinical management of an oft-neglected population. *Pediatrics, 117*(4), 1359–1371.

Kraus, M. F., Susmaras, T., et al. (2007). White matter integrity and cognition in chronic traumatic brain injury: a diffusion tensor imaging study. *Brain, 130*(Pt 10), 2508–2519.

Levine, B., Fujiwara, E., et al. (2006). In vivo characterization of traumatic brain injury neuropathology with structural and functional neuroimaging. *Journal of Neurotrauma, 23*(10), 1396–1411.

Lovell, M. R., Pardini, J. E., et al. (2007). Functional brain abnormalities are related to clinical recovery and time to return to play in athletes. *Neurosurgery, 61*(2), 352–359. discussion 359–360.

Majerske, C. W., Mihalik, J. P., et al. (2008). Concussion in sports: postconcussive activity levels, symptoms, and neurocognitive performance. *Journal of Athletic Training, 43*(3), 265–274.

McAllister, T. W., Flashman, L. A., et al. (2006). Mechanisms of working memory dysfunction after mild and moderate TBI: evidence from functional MRI and neurogenetics. *Journal of Neurotrauma, 23*(10), 1450–1467.

McAllister, T. W., Saykin, A. J., et al. (1999). Brain activation during working memory 1 month after mild traumatic brain injury: a functional MRI study. *Neurology, 53*(6), 1300–1308.

McAllister, T. W., Sparling, M. B., et al. (2001). Differential working memory load effects after mild traumatic brain injury. *NeuroImage, 14*(5), 1004–1012.

McCaffrey, M. A., Mihalik, J. P., et al. (2006). Balance and neurocognitive performance in collegiate football players following head impacts at varying magnitudes. *Journal of Athletic Training, 41*(2), S41.

McCrea, M., Iverson, G. L., et al. (2009). An integrated review of recovery after mild traumatic brain injury (MTBI): Implications for clinical management. *The Clinical Neuropsychologist, 23*(8), 1368–1390.

McCrory, P. (2001). Does second impact syndrome exist? *Clinical Journal of Sport Medicine, 11*(3), 144–149.

McCrory, P., Johnston, K. M., et al. (2001). Evidence-based review of sport-related concussion: basic science. *Clinical Journal of Sport Medicine, 11*(3), 160–165.

McCrory, P., Johnston, K., et al. (2005). Summary and agreement statement of the 2nd International Conference on Concussion in Sport, Prague 2004. *British Journal of Sports Medicine, 39*(4), 196–204.

McCrory, P., Meeuwisse, W., et al. (2009). Consensus Statement on Concussion in Sport: the 3 rd International Conference on Concussion in Sport held in Zurich, November 2008. *British Journal of Sports Medicine, 43*(Suppl 1), i76–i90.

McGowan, J. C., Yang, J. H., et al. (2000). Magnetization transfer imaging in the detection of injury associated with mild head trauma. *American Journal of Neuroradiology, 21*(5), 875–880.

McIntosh, T. K. (1993). Novel pharmacologic therapies in the treatment of experimental traumatic brain injury: a review. *Journal of Neurotrauma, 10*(3), 215–261.

Mihalik, J. P., Guskiewicz, K., et al. (2005). Measurement of head impacts in Division I collegiate football players. *Journal of Athletic Training, 40*(2), S82.

Mihalik, J. P., Guskiewicz, K., et al. (2006). Evaluation of impact biomechanics: the association between impact magnitudes and locations in collegiate football players. *Journal of Athletic Training, 41*(2), S40–S41.

Mussack, T., Biberthaler, P., et al. (2002a). Immediate S-100B and neuron-specific enolase plasma measurements for rapid evaluation of primary brain damage in alcohol-intoxicated, minor head-injured patients. *Shock, 18*(5), 395–400.

Mussack, T., Biberthaler, P., et al. (2002b). Serum S-100B and interleukin-8 as predictive markers for comparative neurologic outcome analysis of patients after cardiac arrest and severe traumatic brain injury. *Critical Care Medicine, 30*(12), 2669–2674.

Myers, R. E. (1979). A unitary theory of causation of anoxic and hypoxic brain pathology. *Advances in Neurology, 26*, 195–213.

Naunheim, R. S., Standeven, J., et al. (2000). Comparison of impact data in hockey, football, and soccer. *The Journal of Trauma, 48*(5), 938–941.

Newman, J. A., Barr, C., et al. (2000). *A new biomechanical assessment of mild traumatic brain injury, Part 2: Results and conclusions.* Montpellier, France: Proceedings of International Research Conference on the Biomechanics of Impacts.

Newman, J. A., Beusenberg, M., et al. (1999). *A new biomechanical assessment of mild traumatic brain injury, Part 1: Methodology.* Barcelona, Spain: Proceedings of International Research Conference on the Biomechanics of Impacts.

Niogi, S. N., Mukherjee, P., et al. (2008a). Extent of microstructural white matter injury in post-concussive syndrome correlates with impaired cognitive reaction time: a 3 T diffusion tensor imaging study of mild traumatic brain injury. *American Journal of Neuroradiology, 29*(5), 967–973.

Niogi, S. N., Mukherjee, P., et al. (2008b). Structural dissociation of attentional control and memory in adults with and without mild traumatic brain injury. *Brain, 131*(Pt 12), 3209–3221.

Ommaya, A. K., & Gennarelli, T. A. (1974). Cerebral concussion and traumatic unconsciousness. Correlation of experimental and clinical observations of blunt head injuries. *Brain, 97*(4), 633–654.

Ommaya, A. K., Gennarelli, T. A., et al. (1973). *Traumatic unconsciousness: mechanisms of brain injury in violent shaking of the head.* Los Angeles, CA: Proceedings of the American Association of Neurological Surgeons.

Ommaya, A. K., Goldsmith, W., et al. (2002). Biomechanics and neuropathology of adult and paediatric head injury. *British Journal of Neurosurgery, 16*(3), 220–242.

Oppenheimer, D. R. (1968). Microscopic lesions in the brain following head injury. *Journal of Neurology, Neurosurgery, and Psychiatry, 31*(4), 299–306.

Osteen, C. L., Moore, A. H., et al. (2001). Age-dependency of 45calcium accumulation following lateral fluid percussion: acute and delayed patterns. *Journal of Neurotrauma, 18*(2), 141–162.

Pellman, E. J. (2003). Background on the National Football League's research on concussion in professional football. *Neurosurgery, 53*(4), 797–798.

Pellman, E. J., Viano, D. C., et al. (2003a). Concussion in professional football: location and direction of helmet impacts-Part 2. *Neurosurgery, 53*(6), 1328–1340. discussion 1340–1341.

Pellman, E. J., Viano, D. C., et al. (2003b). Concussion in professional football: reconstruction of game impacts and injuries. *Neurosurgery, 53*(4), 799–812. discussion 812–814.

Prins, M. L., & Hovda, D. A. (2003). Developing experimental models to address traumatic brain injury in children. *Journal of Neurotrauma, 20*(2), 123–137.

Raghupathi, R. (2004). Cell death mechanisms following traumatic brain injury. *Brain Pathology, 14*(2), 215–222.

Sanders, M. J., Sick, T. J., et al. (2000). Chronic failure in the maintenance of long-term potentiation following fluid percussion injury in the rat. *Brain Research, 861*(1), 69–76.

Schmidt, R. H., & Grady, M. S. (1995). Loss of forebrain cholinergic neurons following fluid-percussion injury: implications for cognitive impairment in closed head injury. *Journal of Neurosurgery, 83*(3), 496–502.

Shaw, N. A. (2002). The neurophysiology of concussion. *Progress in Neurobiology, 67*(4), 281–344.

Sick, T. J., Perez-Pinzon, M. A., et al. (1998). Impaired expression of long-term potentiation in hippocampal slices 4 and 48 h following mild fluid-percussion brain injury in vivo. *Brain Research, 785*(2), 287–292.

Siemkowicz, E., & Hansen, A. J. (1978). Clinical restitution following cerebral ischemia in hypo-, normo- and hyperglycemic rats. *Acta Neurologica Scandinavica, 58*(1), 1–8.

Thibault, K. L., & Margulies, S. S. (1998). Age-dependent material properties of the porcine cerebrum: effect on pediatric inertial head injury criteria. *Journal of Biomechanics, 31*(12), 1119–1126.

Ucar, T., Tanriover, G., et al. (2006). Modified experimental mild traumatic brain injury model. *The Journal of Trauma, 60*(3), 558–565.

Vink, R., Faden, A. I., et al. (1988). Changes in cellular bioenergetic state following graded traumatic brain injury in rats: determination by phosphorus 31 magnetic resonance spectroscopy. *Journal of Neurotrauma, 5*(4), 315–330.

Vink, R., & McIntosh, T. K. (1990). Pharmacological and physiological effects of magnesium on experimental traumatic brain injury. *Magnesium Research, 3*(3), 163–169.

Vink, R., McIntosh, T. K., et al. (1987a). Decrease in total and free magnesium concentration following traumatic brain injury in rats. *Biochemical and Biophysical Research Communications, 149*(2), 594–599.

Vink, R., McIntosh, T. K., et al. (1987b). Effects of traumatic brain injury on cerebral high-energy phosphates and pH: a 31P magnetic resonance spectroscopy study. *Journal of Cerebral Blood Flow and Metabolism, 7*(5), 563–571.

Voller, B., Auff, E., et al. (2001). To do or not to do? Magnetic resonance imaging in mild traumatic brain injury. *Brain Injury, 15*(2), 107–115.

Yarnell, P. R., & Lynch, S. (1970). Retrograde memory immediately after concussion. *The Lancet, 1*(7652), 863–864.

Yarnell, P. R., & Lynch, S. (1973). The 'ding': amnestic states in football trauma. *Neurology, 23*(2), 196–197.

Yoshino, A., Hovda, D. A., et al. (1991). Dynamic changes in local cerebral glucose utilization following cerebral conclusion in rats: evidence of a hyper- and subsequent hypometabolic state. *Brain Research, 561*(1), 106–119.

Zhang, L., Yang, K. H., et al. (2004). A proposed injury threshold for mild traumatic brain injury. *Journal of Biomechanical Engineering, 126*(2), 226–236.

Part II
Assessment and Treatment of Concussion

Chapter 5
Immediate "On-the-Field" Assessment of Concussion

Susannah M. Briskin and Amanda K. Weiss Kelly

5.1 Introduction

This chapter reviews the immediate management of concussion by the sideline medical professional and return to play decision making for the team physician. We outline the use of symptom assessment, physical exam, and neuropsychological testing in the diagnosis and management of concussion. We also provide information on how to perform a complete physical assessment of the concussed athlete and know the uses of sideline and computerized neurological testing in the initial assessment and management of the injured athlete in order to be able to recognize symptoms that would prompt transfer of the injured athlete for hospital evaluation.

As noted in earlier chapters, concussion is defined based on the International Symposia on Concussion in Sport (CIS). The First International Conference on CIS, held in Vienna in 2001, defined concussion as "a complex pathophysiological process affecting the brain, induced by traumatic biomechanical forces." Subsequent CIS meetings in Prague (2004) and Zurich (2008) have maintained this definition (Aubry et al. 2002; McCrory et al. 2005, 2009).

On-the-field assessment of an athlete with suspected concussion involves several distinct key steps. The evaluation starts with the primary survey, including an assessment of the airway, breathing, circulation, and level of consciousness. Next is evaluation of the cervical spine to determine whether the athlete can be safely removed from the playing field to continue the assessment on the sideline or whether he/she should be transported by EMS for emergent evaluation.

S.M. Briskin (✉) • A.K. Weiss Kelly
Rainbow Babies and Children's Hospital, University Hospitals Case Medical Center, Cleveland, OH, USA
e-mail: susannah.briskin@uhhospitals.org; amanda.weiss@uhhospitals.org

J.N. Apps and K.D. Walter (eds.), *Pediatric and Adolescent Concussion:*
Diagnosis, Management and Outcomes, DOI 10.1007/978-0-387-89545-1_5,
© Springer Science+Business Media, LLC 2012

The secondary survey involves a detailed evaluation for concussion, including thorough history, symptom-based survey, comprehensive neurologic examination with cognitive testing, and balance testing. Simple numeric grading of concussion is no longer recommended. Rather, an individualized approach to diagnosis, management, and return to play is standard of practice.

5.2 Primary Survey

The primary survey is the critical starting point with any injured athlete. When an athlete is down on the playing field, the medical team must immediately assess the airway, breathing, and circulation. Rapid assessment to determine the level of consciousness helps further direct appropriate evaluation for concussion and treatment for a possible cervical spine injury.

5.2.1 The Unconscious Athlete

If an injured athlete is unconscious, a cervical spine injury must be presumed and the athlete should not be moved. Proper immobilization of the head and cervical spine by a trained individual is paramount. If CPR is indicated, the chin lift-jaw thrust technique can be used with a helmet and shoulder pads in place and it allows the medical team to open the airway while keeping the cervical spine immobilized. For the athlete who is lying prone, a log roll should be performed to gain access to the injured athlete's airway. This requires several trained medical personnel to adequately protect the cervical spine and turn the patient supine in a coordinated fashion.

There is now universal agreement that protective gear, including helmets and shoulder pads, should not be removed if there is any possibility of a cervical spine injury (Segan et al. 1993; Waninger 1998). Removal of the protective gear used in football and hockey may result in excessive movement of the cervical spine and place the athlete at risk for subsequent injury (Gastel et al. 1998; Metz et al. 1998; LaPrade et al. 2000; Palumbo et al. 1996; Prinsen et al. 1995; Stephensen et al. 1999; Swenson et al. 1997). For sports involving protective headgear, a facemask removal tool (i.e., manual or cordless screwdriver, facemask extractor, trainer's angel) is required to gain adequate access to the airway (Rehberg 1999; Waninger 2004). A trained individual should remove the facemask while the cervical spine is stabilized by a second medical team member (Waninger 2004). This should be performed prior to transport to the emergency room in case the airway must be secured while en route due to patient decompensation.

5.2.2 The Conscious Athlete

For the conscious athlete, it is imperative to evaluate the cervical spine before removing the athlete from the playing field to evaluate for concussion. The injured athlete should be questioned about neck pain, pain radiating into arms/legs, or numbness or tingling in extremities. If any or all of these are present, the cervical spine should be immobilized and the injured athlete should be transported by EMS. If they are absent, then further neurologic assessment should include an evaluation of upper and lower extremity sensation, active range of motion of extremities, and extremity strength. Side-to-side comparison is crucial to detect subtle asymmetry. If any one of these tests is abnormal, the cervical spine should be immobilized and the patient should be transported by EMS. If the athlete remains asymptomatic, palpation of the cervical spine can be performed. Any bony tenderness requires immobilization. If the athlete is nontender, active range of motion of the cervical spine can be performed. If pain free, the athlete can be safely removed from the playing field for formal concussion evaluation. If any sign or symptom warrants cervical immobilization and transportation to the emergency room, no protective gear should be removed, with the exception of the facemask.

An athlete with brief loss of consciousness, defined as less than 1 min, and a normal cervical spine evaluation may be removed from the playing field for comprehensive concussion assessment. It is important to remember that only 10% of individuals who suffer a concussion experience loss of consciousness (Delaney et al. 2002; Guskiewicz et al. 2003; Lovell et al. 1999). Therefore, all athletes who are evaluated for head and/or neck injuries also need evaluation for concussion, regardless of loss of consciousness.

5.3 Secondary Survey

The secondary survey includes a detailed history, comprehensive neurologic exam, cognitive testing, and balance testing. The overall goal is to determine whether signs or symptoms of concussion are present. Establishing a baseline of sign and symptom severity is critical for following the athlete over time to determine further management.

On occasion, athletes who have suffered a concussion do not disclose their symptoms to medical staff due to a fear of being withheld from their sport (McCrea et al. 2004). Some athletes also fear criticism from teammates, parents, or coaches. Thus, it is imperative that the medical team have a high index of suspicion for concussion and look for subtle signs of concussion when evaluating athletes. Also, it is common for teammates or coaches to notice changes in a concussed athlete during a sporting event and bring them to the medical team's attention. These subtle signs include a dazed appearance, confusion about their responsibilities in the game, forgetfulness, poor coordination, behavior or personality changes,

Table 5.1 Common signs and symptoms of concussion

Physical	Cognitive	Emotional	Sleep related
Headache	Mentally "foggy"	Irritable	Drowsiness
Nausea	Feeling slowed down	Sadness	Sleep more than usual
Vomiting	Difficulty concentrating	Emotional liability	Sleep less than usual
Balance problems	Difficulty remembering	Nervousness or anxiousness	Difficulty falling asleep
Dizziness	Forgetfulness		
Visual problems	Confusion		
Fatigue	Slow to answer questions		
Sensitivity to light	Repeats questions		
Sensitivity to noise			
Numbness/tingling			
Loss of consciousness			
Amnesia			
Dazed			
Stunned			

inability to remember events, witnessed brief loss of consciousness, and slow response to questions (Lovell 2009). An athlete displaying even a single sign or symptom of concussion requires further evaluation.

Sideline evaluation begins with a detailed history surrounding the injury. Mechanism and timing of injury are important. However, an injured athlete may not be able to provide this information if amnesia is present. Sometimes parents, teammates, or coaches can provide more detailed information about the situation to assist the medical team.

Assessment of signs and symptoms is crucial not only in making a diagnosis of concussion, but also for establishing a baseline to follow. Signs and symptoms can be separated into four categories: physical, cognitive, emotional, and sleep related (US Department of Health and Human Services and Center for Disease Control and Prevention 2010) (Table 5.1). Headaches are the most commonly reported symptom (Blinman et al. 2009). Loss of consciousness for greater than 30 s, significant amnesia, or worsening headache is an indicator of a potentially more serious head injury, such as an intracranial bleed (Collins et al. 2003; Kelly 2001; Guskiewicz et al. 2000b). Emergent evaluation with advanced imaging should be strongly considered when any of these are present.

Objective documentation of concussion signs and symptoms is best achieved using a standardized postconcussion scale. The Pittsburgh Steelers Postconcussion Scale developed in the 1980s was the first of its kind (Maroon et al. 2000). It utilized a 17-item questionnaire to document symptoms on the sidelines. Grading of symptoms was documented on a 7-point Likert scale (Table 5.2).

Many concussion scales have been developed utilizing the Pittsburgh Steeler's Postconcussion Scale as a model. The majority of these use a Likert scale to document a wide breadth of concussion signs and symptoms. Most of the popular scales

Table 5.2 Postconcussion symptom scale

Symptom	Score						
	0---------------------3------------------6						
	None		Moderate			Severe	
Headache	0	1	2	3	4	5	6
Nausea	0	1	2	3	4	5	6
Vomiting	0	1	2	3	4	5	6
Balance problems	0	1	2	3	4	5	6
Dizziness	0	1	2	3	4	5	6
Fatigue	0	1	2	3	4	5	6
Trouble falling to sleep	0	1	2	3	4	5	6
Excessive sleep	0	1	2	3	4	5	6
Loss of sleep	0	1	2	3	4	5	6
Drowsiness	0	1	2	3	4	5	6
Light sensitivity	0	1	2	3	4	5	6
Noise sensitivity	0	1	2	3	4	5	6
Irritability	0	1	2	3	4	5	6
Sadness	0	1	2	3	4	5	6
Nervousness	0	1	2	3	4	5	6
More emotional	0	1	2	3	4	5	6
Numbness	0	1	2	3	4	5	6
Feeling "slow"	0	1	2	3	4	5	6
Feeling "foggy"	0	1	2	3	4	5	6
Difficulty concentrating	0	1	2	3	4	5	6
Difficulty remembering	0	1	2	3	4	5	6
Visual problems	0	1	2	3	4	5	6

score about 20 signs and symptoms. Unfortunately, little scientific research has been done to document their reliability (Alla et al. 2009; Gioia et al. 2009).

Recent data does demonstrate significant correlations between symptoms reported on the Postconcussion Symptom Scale with neuropsychological deficits and postural stability deficits (Broglio and Guskiewicz 2009). Specifically, feeling "dizziness" or reporting "balance problems" was correlated to balance deficits on the Sensory Organization Test. "Feeling mentally foggy" was related to decreased reaction time on ImPACT testing. Finally, "difficulty concentrating" was correlated with verbal memory score and "difficulty remembering" was related to verbal memory score and reaction time. Also, as the athlete reported worsening symptom severity, greater declines in performance on clinical tests were noted. These correlations support the validity of the symptom scale in assessing true cognitive and postural deficits. It also demonstrates the athlete's ability to accurately identify concussion-related impairments and supports the use of a multifaceted approach to concussion diagnosis and management. If the athlete is unable or unwilling to provide an accurate account of symptoms, clinical tests, such as balance testing or cognitive testing, can provide alternative evidence of impairment.

These scales are subjective measures, and are therefore dependent not only on the athlete's own insight but also his/her honesty (Piland et al. 2003; Van Kampen et al. 2006; McCrea et al. 2004; Broglio and Puetz 2008). Recent research suggests that as many as 10% of athletes may underreport concussion symptoms (Broglio and Guskiewicz 2009; McCrea et al. 2004). This supports the use of objective measures of concussion, such as postural and cognitive testing, in addition to symptom reporting in the management of concussion.

A recent investigation highlights the importance of obtaining a baseline assessment of symptoms. Shehata et al. demonstrated that the mean preinjury baseline total symptom score on the Postconcussion Symptom Scale was 4.29 (Shehata et al. 2009). The symptoms most commonly reported were fatigue, drowsiness, neck pain, difficulty concentrating, and difficulty remembering. This demonstrates that some level of symptomatology can be expected at baseline, so postinjury results should be interpreted in the context of the athlete's individual baseline score.

Finally, these symptom scales may also not be appropriate for school-aged athletes, as little research has been done to assess their validity in this population (Gioia et al. 2009).

The future of concussion documentation on the field will be geared toward improving the concussion signs and symptoms checklists. The checklists will likely undergo scientific scrutiny as individuals look to identify the key diagnostic features and prove reliability and validity.

The comprehensive physical exam includes several key components: head and neck exam, complete neurological exam, cognitive testing which can be done using the Sport Concussion Assessment Tool 2 (SCAT2) and Balance-Error Scoring System (BESS) testing. The first step of the physical exam includes an evaluation for facial trauma. This is especially important in sports where helmets are not worn. Observation for facial symmetry and documentation of swelling or bruising is important. Palpation of facial bones for tenderness or crepitus should be performed. Evaluation for dental injuries includes an assessment of jaw alignment. The neurologic exam begins with evaluation of extraocular eye movements, pupillary response to light, and fundoscopic exam. Cranial nerve exam, sensation testing, upper and lower extremity strength testing, reflexes, and cerebellar testing should all be performed.

5.4 On-Field Cognitive Testing

While concussion is easily recognized in the athlete who suffers loss of consciousness or significant disorientation after a head injury, many athletes have more subtle symptoms. Historically, physicians have used many different methods of assessing mental status after head injury, including counting backward by increments, reciting the months of the year in reverse order, and remembering lists of words (McCrea 2001a, b). The lack of standardization and increasing acknowledgment of the importance of appropriate recognition and management of sport-related concussion have spurred a movement to develop standardized cognitive testing to aide in the sideline diagnosis and management of concussion.

Table 5.3 Traditional orientation questions, Maddocks et al. (1995)

- What is your name?
- What is your date of birth?
- How old are you?
- What year is it?
- What month is it?
- What day of the week is it?
- What is the date?
- What time of day is it – morning, afternoon, or night?

Table 5.4 Maddocks questions, Maddocks et al. (1995)

- At which ground are we?
- Which quarter is it?
- How far into the quarter is it – the first, middle, or last 10 min?
- Which side kicked the last goal?
- Which team did we play last week?
- Did we win last week?

Early research recognized that the traditional cognitive assessment of orientation to time, person, and place used to assess victims of motor vehicle collisions is not sensitive enough to recognize concussion in athletes with head injury, since athletes' injuries are sustained with significantly less force than victims of motor vehicle collisions. In 1995, Maddocks et al. investigated the sensitivity of traditional orientation items (Table 5.3) compared to questions relating to recently acquired information in athletes with head injury (Maddocks et al. 1995). They discovered that athletes with concussion had significantly more difficulty answering questions related to recent memory (see Table 5.4) than controls. Injured athletes and controls did not differ in their ability to answer traditional orientation questions.

Later efforts, such as those by McCrea et al., attempted to standardize the cognitive exam using the Standardized Assessment of Concussion (SAC) test (McCrea et al. 1997). The SAC includes four domains of cognitive function: orientation, immediate memory, concentration, and recall. In the initial study to establish reliability and validity, athletes were tested prior to the season to establish a baseline and then, again, immediately after concussion. Also, matched uninjured controls were tested at the same time periods. In addition to establishing the reliability and validity of the SAC in discriminating athletes with mild concussion from uninjured athletes, they also demonstrated the feasibility of using the SAC as part of the sideline exam in collegiate football players. A later investigation using the SAC test evaluated athletes suffering concussion with a baseline, immediate postinjury assessment, and 48-h assessment (McCrea et al. 1998). Players suffering from concussion scored an average of 3.5 points lower than baseline, 1.48 standard deviations below baseline, and 1.58 standard deviations below the mean for the control group. These findings were particularly significant since none of the injured players were obviously disoriented or neurologically impaired, demonstrating that the SAC could identify subtle cognitive changes in the athlete with concussion despite the lack of other obvious symptoms. All injured athletes in this study returned to baseline within 48 h. Further investigation demonstrated that a drop of one point or more from preseason baseline on the SAC test was 95% sensitive and 76% specific in correctly classifying injured and uninjured athletes (McCrea 2001a, b). These studies support the reliability and validity of the SAC in detecting mental status change occurring as a result of concussion.

Another group investigated the utility of the SAC test in collegiate football and soccer players. This study demonstrated the reliability of the SAC as an objective measure of assessing cognitive changes associated with concussion. However, a significant portion, 50%, of injured athletes were still symptomatic at the time that their SAC score returned to baseline, making the utility of using SAC testing in guiding return to play decisions questionable (Hecht et al. 2004). This group also demonstrated a learning effect, with the control players' SAC scores increasing with retesting and 29% of concussed players scoring greater than baseline on the day of concussion.

The SAC provides an excellent gross-level measure of mental status in the athlete with concussion and is a very useful part of the sideline exam. However, it is intended to be used along with physical exam and other signs of injury in the assessment of concussion. It is not intended to replace formal neurologic or neuropsychological evaluation. As SAC scores may return to normal before the resolution of symptoms, it is also not intended for use in return to play decision making.

The SCAT is a standardized method of evaluating athletes suspected of concussion that was developed and produced as part of the 2004 Prague CIS International Conference (McCrory et al. 2005). It includes a symptom checklist, Maddocks questions, the SAC test, and neurologic screening. The SCAT2 was introduced by the third CIS, adding the Glasgow coma scale, postural stability assessment, and coordination exam (McCrory et al. 2009).

As mentioned earlier, a recent investigation highlights the correlation between deficits on neuropsychological testing and self-reported symptoms on the postconcussion symptom checklist (Broglio and Guskiewicz 2009). Thus, sideline cognitive testing may be particularly useful when it is suspected that an athlete may be underreporting symptoms and reinforces the importance of using the entire history and exam and not just one component in the assessment concussion.

5.5 Current Research Involving the Balance-Error Scoring System

The use of postural and stability testing in the assessment of concussion was intended to provide objective information regarding the athlete with suspected concussion. Investigators have tested postural stability after head injury using force plates, which are impractical for sideline assessment, and clinical measures of balance without use of a force plate, which are much more easily replicated on the sidelines (Riemann and Guskiewicz 2000; Guskiewicz et al. 2001).

Table 5.5 Balance-error scoring system errors, Riemann et al. (1999)

- Lifting hands off of the iliac crests
- Opening eyes
- Stepping, stumbling, or falling
- Flexing or abducting hip more than 30°
- Lifting the forefoot or heel
- Remaining out of the testing position for more than 5 s

Early research demonstrating that head injury can cause axonal dysfunction at the level of the brainstem or cerebellum, areas that can affect balance, led researchers to begin to use balance testing in the evaluation of concussion (Guskiewicz et al. 2000a). The earliest test used to assess balance in the head-injured athlete was the Romberg test. The need for a more challenging and detailed assessment with better sensitivity and specificity led to the use of force plates to assess balance. Using force plate testing, investigators demonstrated that changes in postural stability persisted for up to 3–5 days after concussion. The greatest differences between subjects and controls were noted when visual cues were removed or the support surface was changed (Guskiewicz et al. 1997; McCrea et al. 2003).

The impracticality of using force plate balance testing in sideline decision making led to the development of detailed clinical balance scoring systems, including the BESS. BESS has been shown to correlate well with force-platform sway measures (Riemann et al. 1999). In BESS testing, the athlete performs three different stances: the double-leg stance, single-leg stance, and tandem stance, first on a firm surface and then on a 2.5-in.-thick foam surface with hands on hips. The subject is asked to hold each stance for 20 s. One point is scored for every error made (see Table 5.5). If the athlete stumbles out of position, timing is stopped and then started again once the testing stance is resumed. Testing on a foam surface reveals more significant differences compared to controls than testing on a firm surface (Riemann and Guskiewicz 2000). Having three or more errors compared to baseline has sensitivity for concussion diagnosis of 34% and a specificity of 91% (McCrea et al. 2005).

BESS testing scores return to normal, compared to individual baseline testing, at the same time that symptoms related to concussion resolve, except for headache, which some athletes continued to complain of for several days after BESS testing returns to normal (Guskiewicz et al. 2001; Riemann and Guskiewicz 2000 JAT). Loss of consciousness does not seem to influence how quickly BESS testing returns to baseline, reinforcing the idea that LOC should not be a central marker for severity of concussion (Guskiewicz et al. 2001). BESS testing is a valid and reliable method of testing postural stability after concussion that is inexpensive and easy to use on the sidelines or in the training room. Although its ratio of sensitivity to specificity means that normal findings should not be interpreted to suggest the absence of concussion, positive findings are more likely to be meaningful.

On the other hand, more recent research of BESS testing demonstrated that normal subjects, without head injury, have a significantly increased number of errors on BESS testing immediately after fatiguing exercise compared to baseline and controls (Crowell et al. 2001; Wilkins et al. 2004; Susco et al. 2004). Investigators have demonstrated that the effects of fatigue on postural stability seem to resolve after 15–20 min of rest in tests using both force plate and BESS (Susco et al. 2004; Nardone et al. 1998). Thus, BESS administration may provide more relevant information after an injured athlete has had 15–20 min to rest.

One recent study demonstrated improved reliability of BESS testing by removing the double-leg stance portion and performing three trials of the single-leg and tandem stance on a firm surface and foam surface without affecting efficiency or convenience (Hunt et al. 2009).

Another recent investigation demonstrated the correlation between postural stability and complaints of "balance problems" on the postconcussion symptom checklist, highlighting the relationship between symptoms and objective clinical measures of balance and the usefulness of a multifaceted approach to concussion diagnosis (Broglio and Guskiewicz 2009).

In the future, the use of a standardized sideline assessment of concussion that evaluates multiple dimensions of mental status, including orientation, immediate memory, delayed recall, and concentration, in conjunction with physical exam and postural, coordination, and symptom assessment will be commonplace. The complete assessment of the athlete should take each of these individual tests into consideration.

While there is excellent data regarding the validity, reliability, sensitivity, and specificity of the SAC test in highschool and collegiate athletes, there is no data available regarding these same measures in the SCAT or SCAT2. While it has been suggested by the CIS group that the SCAT2 can be used in athletes older than 10 years of age, data regarding the use of cognitive testing in pre-highschool athletes is limited. Further investigation in young athletes is warranted to determine typical baseline scores, scores after concussion, and time to return to baseline after injury in this age group. Furthermore, no standardized testing for athletes younger than the age of 10 has been offered at all. Attempts to study concussion and develop tools for concussion assessment in this age group is essential (McCrory et al. 2009). Since the bulk of postural testing has been performed with college age, Division I NCAA athletes, BESS testing in the teen and preteen age groups offers more specific information regarding balance assessment after head injury in the pediatric age group.

5.6 Grading

More than 25 different concussion grading systems have been developed (Johnston et al. 2001), and this topic was covered extensively in Chapter 2 of this book. Previously, the three most commonly referenced grading systems were the American Academy of Neurology (AAN), Colorado Medical Society (CMS), and the Cantu Grading System. These systems based their concussion grading upon loss of consciousness, presence of amnesia, and duration of symptoms. The grade of the concussion was subsequently used to classify athletes and guide their return to play (Practice Parameter: The Management of Concussion in Sports Summary Statement 1997; Society CM 1991; Cantu 1986, 2001).

The 2001 Vienna CIS acknowledged the widespread use of the grading systems and commented on their individual strengths and weaknesses. A formal recommendation was made to abandon the grading systems, and a new approach aimed at delineating each individual athlete's injury severity was endorsed. This marked the beginning of the movement toward individualized return to play guidelines (Aubry et al. 2002).

The 2004 Prague CIS made a brief return to categorizing athletes as they coined the new terms of "simple" and "complex" concussion. A "simple" concussion was defined as an injury with symptoms that progressively resolved within 7–10 days. A "complex" concussion was defined by an injury with symptoms persisting beyond 10 days or when any of the following were present: LOC > 1 min, postconcussive seizure, or prolonged cognitive impairment resulted after the concussion. Also, individuals who suffered multiple concussions over time or those athletes who sustained concussions after lower amounts of force were considered "complex." The purpose of the "simple" and "complex" categorization was to aid in management recommendations of athletes who suffer concussion. However, this new classification system was not practical for on-the-field management since athletes could not be categorized in most cases until after their symptoms resolved (McCrory et al. 2005).

The 2008 Zurich CIS no longer endorsed grading systems or even categorization into "simple" and "complex" concussions. Rather, the conference formally recommended a comprehensive individual assessment of each athlete with return to play decisions based upon each individual's resolution of signs and symptoms (McCrory et al. 2009).

5.7 Immediate Management of Concussion by Sideline Medical Professional

While no longer an accepted practice, early concussion management endorsed return to play in the same contest if the athlete was without symptoms 15 min after injury (Johnston et al. 2001). Recent evidence demonstrates that symptoms may develop or worsen after the initial assessment at the time of injury (Echemendia et al. 2001). Lovell et al. demonstrated that highschool athletes' self-reported symptoms and memory as tested with ImPACT testing worsened for up to 36 h after mild injury, which would have previously been classified as grade I concussion, allowing for a potential same-day return to play (Lovell et al. 2004). This propensity for symptoms to develop and progress after the initial assessment highlights the importance of restricting play as soon as injury is recognized and continued monitoring of

Table 5.6 Criteria for hospital transport from sidelines, Osmond et al. (2010)

- Potential cervical spine injury
- Deterioration in mental status
- Focal neurological symptoms
- Prolonged loss of consciousness
- Severe headache
- Recurrent emesis
- Glasgow Coma Scale less than 15
- Suspected skull fracture
- Suspected basal skull fracture (hemotympanum, "raccoon" eyes, otorrhea, rhinorrhea or cerebrospinal fluid, Battle's sign)
- Large boggy scalp hematoma

the athlete with suspected concussion. It also supports the recent recommendations to not allow same-day return to play when concussion is diagnosed, especially in the pediatric athlete (McCrory et al. 2009). Many organizations use the tagline, "When in Doubt, Sit Them Out!"

Historical management, which remains relevant today, suggests that all athletes with signs or symptoms that suggest intracranial bleed should be transported to the hospital immediately (see Table 5.6) (Osmond et al. 2010).

Because athletes may unknowingly or purposefully underreport concussive symptoms, the use of a multifaceted approach to concussion diagnosis and management that includes objective measures of postural stability and cognitive impairment, in addition to symptom reporting, is essential.

5.8 Monitoring and Management During the First 24 Hours After Injury

It is important for the athlete, coach, parents, and roommates to understand what to look for in the athlete with a concussion. If any of the signs of worsening mental status (see Table 5.7) develop after leaving the care of the sideline physician, the athlete should be transported to the hospital. The athlete with concussion should not be left alone, as symptoms may rapidly worsen. Concussed athletes should be considered unsafe for driving until cleared by a physician.

Clear follow-up instructions for reevaluation by medical staff should be provided before allowing the athlete to leave the field. Ideally, these instructions are discussed with the athlete and the athlete's parents or primary care giver. Typically, follow-up the next day is recommended, whenever possible.

Table 5.7 Criteria for hospital evaluation, McCrory et al. (2009)

- Worsening headache
- Athlete is very drowsy or cannot be awakened
- Inability to recognize people or places
- Repeated emesis
- Unusual or very irritable behavior
- Seizures
- Weakness
- Unsteady gait

5.9 Summary

Evaluation of concussion has moved away from an emphasis on the grading of injury and toward early recognition and individualized assessment of concussion signs and symptoms. These can be easily documented using a Likert scale that can be performed after injury to follow injured athletes over time. Comprehensive sideline evaluation should also include cognitive assessment and balance testing. No athlete with a concussion should be allowed to return to play the same day of the injury. Athletes should not be allowed to return to play if they are still experiencing symptoms. Every athlete should receive medical clearance from a health care provider prior to returning to sport.

5.10 Key Points

Evaluation of the cervical spine is crucial in an injured athlete.

Loss of consciousness occurs in only 10% of concussions.

Diagnosis of a concussion requires that only a single sign or symptom of concussion be present.

Use of a Postconcussion Symptom Scale before injury helps establish a baseline which can be used in context to assess symptoms after injury.

Sideline concussion evaluation should be multifaceted and include a complete neurologic exam, cognitive testing, and balance tests.

Grading scales for concussion are no longer utilized.

Adolescent athletes commonly have worsening of symptoms in the first 48 hours after injury.

Any athlete who is diagnosed with a concussion should not return to play the same day.

References

Alla, S., Sullivan, S. J., Hale, L., et al. (2009). Self-report scales/checklists for the measurement of concussion symptoms: a systematic review. *British Journal of Sports Medicine, 43*(Suppl. 1), i3–i12.

Aubry, M., Cantu, R., Dvorak, J., et al. (2002). Summary and agreement statement of the 1st International Symposium on Concussion in Sport: Vienna 2001. *Clinical Journal of Sport Medicine, 12*, 6–11.

Blinman, T. A., Houseknecht, E., Snyder, C., et al. (2009). Postconcussive symptoms in hospitalized pediatric patients after mild traumatic brain injury. *Journal of Pediatric Surgery, 44*, 1223–1228.

Broglio, S. P., & Guskiewicz, K. M. (2009). Concussion in sports: the sideline assessment. *Sports Health, 1*, 361–369.

Broglio, S., & Puetz, T. (2008). The effect of sports concussion on neurocognitive function, self-report symptoms and postural control: a meta-analysis. *Sports Medicine, 38*, 53–67.

Cantu, R. C. (1986). Guidelines for return to contact sports after cerebral concussion. *The Physician and Sportsmedicine, 14*, 75–83.

Cantu, R. C. (2001). Posttraumatic retrograde and anterograde amnesia: pathophysiology and implications in grading and safe return to play. *Journal of Athletic Training, 36*, 249–252.

Collins, M. W., Iverson, G., et al. (2003). On-field predictors of neuropsychological and symptom deficit following sports-related concussion. *Clin J Sports Med, 13*(4), 222–229.

Crowell, D. H., Guskeiwicz, K. M., Prentice, W. E., & Onate, J. A. (2001). The effect of fatigue on postural stability and neuropsycholoical function (abstrct). *Journal of Athletic Training, 36*, S33.

Delaney, J. S., Lacroix, V. J., Leclerc, S., & Johnson, K. M. (2002). Concussions among university football and soccer players. *Clinical Journal of Sport Medicine, 12*(6), 331–338.

Echemendia, R. L., Putukian, M., Mackin, R. S., et al. (2001). Neuropsychological test performance prior to and following sports-related mild traumatic brain injury. *Clinical Journal of Sport Medicine, 11*, 23–31.

Gastel, J. A., Palumbo, M. A., Hulstyn, M. J., et al. (1998). Emergency removal of football equipment: a cadaveric cervical spine injury model. *Annals of Emergency Medicine, 32*, 411–417.

Gioia, G. A., Schneider, J. C., Vaughan, C. G., et al. (2009). Which symptom assessments and approaches are uniquely appropriate for paediatric concussion? *British Journal of Sports Medicine, 43*, i13–i22.

Guskiewicz, K. M., McCrea, M., Marshall, S. W., et al. (2003). Cumulative effects associated with recurrent concussion in collegiate football players: the NCAA concussion study. *Journal of American Medical Association, 290*(19), 2549–2555.

Guskiewicz, K. M., Perrin, D. H., & Gansneder, B. M. (2000a). Effects of mild head injury on postural stability in athletes. *Journal of Athletic Training, 35*, 19–25.

Guskiewicz, K. M., Riemann, B. L., Perrin, D. H., & Nasher, L. M. (1997). Alternative approaches to the assessment of mild head injury in athletes. *Medicine and Science in Sports and Exercise, 29*, S213–S221.

Guskiewicz, K. M., Ross, S. E., & Marshall, S. W. (2001). Postural stability and neuropsychological deficits after cuncussion in collegiate athletes. *Journal of Athletic Training, 36*, 263–273.

Guskiewicz, K. M., Weaver, N. L., Padua, D. A., & Garrett, W. E. (2000b). Epidemiology of concussion in collegiate and high school football players. *The American Journal of Sports Medicine, 28*, 643–650.

Hecht, S., Puffer, J., Clinton, C., Aish, B., Cohen, P., Concoff, A., et al. (2004). Concussion assessment in football and soccer players. *Clinical Journal of Sport Medicine, 14*, 310.

Hunt, T., Ferrara, M. S., Bornstein, R. A., & Baumgartner, T. A. (2009). The reliability of the modified balance error scoring system. *Clinical Journal of Sport Medicine, 19*, 471–475.

Johnston, K. M., McCrory, P., Mohtadi, N., & Meeuwisse, W. (2001). Evidence-based review of sport-related concussion: clinical science. *Clinical Journal of Sport Medicine, 11*, 150–159.

Kelly, J. (2001). Loss of consciousness: pathophysiology and implications in grading and safe return to play. *Journal of Athletic Training, 36*, 249–252.

LaPrade, R. F., Schnetzler, K., Boxterman, R. J., et al. (2000). Cervical spine alignment in the immobilized ice hockey player: a computed tomographic analysis of the effects of helmet removal. *The American Journal of Sports Medicine, 28*, 800–803.

Lovell, M. (2009). The management of sports-related concussion: current status and future trends. *Clinics in Sports Medicine, 28*, 95–111.

Lovell, M. R., Collins, M. W., Iverson, G. L., Johnston, K. M., & Bradley, J. P. (2004). Grade 1 or "Ding" concussions in high school athletes. *American Journal of Sports Medicine, 32*, 47–54.

Lovell, M. R., Iverson, G. L., Collins, M. W., McKeag, D. B., & Maroon, J. C. (1999). Does loss of consciousness predict neuropsychological decrements after concussion? *Clinical Journal of Sport Medicine, 9*(4), 193–198.

Maddocks, D. L., Dicker, G. D., & Saling, M. M. (1995). The assessment of orientation following concussion in athletes. *Clinical Journal of Sport Medicine, 5*, 32–35.

Maroon, J., Lovell, M., Norwig, J., et al. (2000). Cerebral concussion in athletes: evaluation and neuropsychological testing. *Neurosurgery, 47*, 659–669. discussion 669–672.

McCrea, M. (2001a). Standardized mental status testing on the sideline after sport-related concussion. *Journal of Athletic Training, 36*, 274–279.

McCrea, M. (2001b). Standardized mental status assessment of concussion. *Clinical Journal of Sport Medicine, 11*, 176–181.

McCrea, M., Burr, W. B., & Guskiewicz, K. (2005). Standard regression-based methods for measuring recovery after sport-related concussion. *Journal of International Neuropsychology Society, 11*, 58–69.

McCrea, M., Guskiewicz, K. M., Marshall, S. W., Barr, W., Randolph, C., Cantu, R., et al. (2003). Acute effects and recovery time following concussion in collegiate football players. The NCAA concussion study. *Journal of American Medical Association, 290*, 2556–2563.

McCrea, M., Hammeke, T., Olsen, G., Leo, P., & Guskiewicz, K. (2004). Unreported concussion in high school football players: implications for prevention. *Clinical Journal of Sport Medicine, 14*(1), 13–17.

McCrea, M., Kelly, J. P., Kluge, J., Ackley, B. A., & Randolph, C. (1997). Standardized assessment of concussion in football players. *Neurology, 48*, 586–588.

McCrea, M., Kelly, J. P., Randolph, C., Kluge, J., Bartolic, E., Finn, G., et al. (1998). Standardized assessment of concussion (SAC): on-site mental status evaluation of the athlete. *The Journal of Head Trauma Rehabilitation, 13*(2), 27–35.

McCrory, P., Johnston, K., Meeuwisse, W., et al. (2005). Summary and agreement statement of the 2nd International Symposium on Concussion in Sport 2004, Prague. *British Journal of Sports Medicine, 39*, 196–204.

McCrory, P., Meeuwisse, W., Johnston, K., et al. (2009). Concensus statement on Concussion in Sport 3rd International Symposium on Concussion in Sport held in Zurich, November 2008. *Clinical Journal of Sports Medicine, 19*(3), 185–200.

Metz, C. M., Kuhn, J. E., & Greenfield, M. L. (1998). Cervical spine alignment in immobilized hockey players: radiographic analysis with and without helmets and shoulder pads. *Clinical Journal of Sport Medicine, 8*, 92–95.

Nardone, A., Tarantola, J., Galante, M., & Schieppati, M. (1998). Time course of stabilometric changes after a strenuous treadmill exercise. *Archives of Physical Medicine and Rehabilitation, 79*, 920–924.

Osmond, M. H., Klasen, T. P., Wells, G. A., Correll, R., Jarvis, A., Joubert, G., et al. (2010). CATCH: a clinical decision rule for the use of computed tomography in children with minor head injury. *Canadian Medical Association Journal.* doi:10.1503/cmaj.091421.

Palumbo, M. A., Hulstyn, M. J., Fadale, P. D., et al. (1996). The effect of protective football equipment on alignment of the injured cervical spine: radiographic analysis in a cadaveric model. *The American Journal of Sports Medicine, 24*, 446–453.

Piland, S., Motl, R., Ferrara, M., et al. (2003). Evidence for the factorial and construct validity of a self-report concussion symptoms scale. *Journal of Athletic Training, 38*, 104–112.

Practice Parameter: the management of concussion in sports (summary statement). (1997). Report of the Quality Standards Subcommittee of the American Academy of Neurology. *Neurology, 48*, 581–585.

Prinsen, R. K. E., Syrotuik, D. G., & Reid, D. C. (1995). Position of the cervical vertebrae during helmet removal and cervical collar application in football and hockey. *Clinical Journal of Sport Medicine, 5*, 155–161.

Rehberg, R. S. (1999). Facemask removal tools come in all shapes, styles. *NATA News, 8*, 8–9.

Riemann, B. L., & Guskiewicz, K. M. (2000). Effects of mild head injury on postural stability as measured through clinical balance testing. *Journal of Athletic Training, 35*, 19–25.

Riemann, B. L., Guskiewicz, K. M., & Shields, E. W. (1999). Relationship between clinical and forecplate measures of postural stability. *Journal of Sport Rehabilitation, 8*, 71–82.

Segan, R. D., Cassidy, C., & Bentkowski, J. (1993). A discussion of the issue of football helmet removal in suspected cervical spine injuries. *Journal of Athletic Training, 28*, 294–305.

Shehata, N., Wiley, J. P., Richea, S., et al. (2009). Sport concussion assessment tool: baseline values for varsity collision sport athletes. *British Journal of Sports Medicine, 43*, 730–734.

Society, C. M. (1991). *Report of the Sports Medicine Committee: Guidelines for the Management of Concussions in Sport (Revised)*. Denver: Colorado Medical society.

Stephensen, A., Horodyski, M. B., Meister, K., et al. (1999). Cervical spine alignment in the immobilized ice hockey player: radiographic analysis before and after helmet removal [abstract]. *Journal of Athletic Training, 34*, S27.

Susco, T. M., Valovich, T. C., Gansneder, B. M., & Shultz, S. J. (2004). Balance recovers within 20 minutes after exertion as measured by the balance error scoring system. *Journal of Athletic Training, 39*, 241–246.

Swenson, T. M., Lauerman, W. C., Donaldson, W. F., et al. (1997). Cervical spine alignment in the immobilized football player: radiographic analysis before and after helmet removal. *The American Journal of Sports Medicine, 25*, 226–230.

US Department of Health and Human Services, Center for Disease Control and Prevention. Heads up: facts for physicians about mild traumatic brain injury (MTBI) (2010) http://www.cdc.gov/concussion/headsup/pdf/Facts_for_Physicians_booklet_a.pdf. Accessed September 23, 2011.

Van Kampen, D., Lovell, M., Pardini, J., et al. (2006). The "value added" of neurocognitive testing after sports-related concussion. *American Journal of Sports Medicine, 34*, 1630–1635.

Waninger, K. N. (1998). On-field management of potential cervical spine injury in helmeted football players: leave the helmet on! *Clinical Journal of Sports Medicine, 8*, 124–129.

Waninger, K. N. (2004). Management of the helmeted athlete with suspected cervical spine injury. *The American Journal of Sports Medicine, 32*, 1331–1350.

Wilkins, J. C., Valovich McLeod, T. C., Perrin, D. H., & Gansneder, B. M. (2004). Performance on the balance error scoring system decreases after fatigue. *Journal of Athletic Training, 39*, 156–161.

Chapter 6
Acute Treatment of Concussion

Danny G. Thomas

6.1   Introduction

An estimated 615,000 TBIs occur each year in patients younger than 19 years old, representing 26% of pediatric hospitalizations and 15% of all pediatric deaths (Langlois et al. 2005; Sosin et al. 1996). Mild Traumatic Brain Injury (mTBI), or concussion, represents the predominant form of acquired brain injury, accounting for 75–90% of all instances (Schultz 2004). Patients with mTBI most often present to the emergency department (ED) or primary care office, neither of which specialize in the diagnosis and treatment of mTBI. Of those patients with mTBI that seek immediate care in the ED, the majority are given reassurance and discharged to their home. In the ED setting, the accurate assessment of injury severity and consequent outpatient guidance and management are critical to ensuring safe recovery from the injury. Appropriate diagnosis, patient education, and outpatient management may decrease recovery time, reduce risk of secondary complications and improve outcomes. Historically, however, the evaluation and management of concussion have been inconsistent, and outcomes are largely unknown. To add to the confusion, over 25 concussion grading systems exist, each with their own ranking of concussion severity and management recommendations. Unfortunately, these clinical grading systems are not validated and have not allowed clinicians, patients, or families to recognize the full spectrum of postconcussive symptoms (AAN 1997; Metzl 2006). Furthermore, the ED setting is unique in its focus on immediate care needs and its inherent limitations with continuity of care. Early identification and diagnosis in this setting is vital to promoting a safe recovery.

D.G. Thomas (✉)
Assistant Professor of Pediatrics, Emergency Medicine,
Medical College of Wisconsin, Milwaukee, WI, USA
e-mail: dthomas@mcw.edu

J.N. Apps and K.D. Walter (eds.), *Pediatric and Adolescent Concussion:
Diagnosis, Management and Outcomes*, DOI 10.1007/978-0-387-89545-1_6,
© Springer Science+Business Media, LLC 2012

This chapter focuses on acute management of the concussed patient, addressing three key issues: (1) identifying those patients with more significant intracranial injury, (2) treating physical symptoms post concussion, and (3) minimizing further secondary injury during the recovery period. This chapter will review the indications for referral to the ED and indications for emergent neuroimaging, management strategies for physical complaints following concussion, and outpatient follow-up strategies to minimize secondary injury.

6.2 Pathology of Head Trauma

mTBI or concussion, in the recent CDC Physician's mTBI Toolkit, is defined as: "(a) complex pathophysiologic process affecting the brain, induced by traumatic biomechanical forces secondary to direct or indirect forces to the head. mTBI is caused by a blow or jolt to the head that disrupts the function of the brain. This disturbance of brain function is typically associated with normal structural neuroimaging findings (i.e., CT scan, MRI) (CDC 2007)." Injuries that cause structural damage to the brain mean the patient has suffered moderate to severe traumatic brain injury. The greater the traumatic force, the greater the injury to brain tissue. Head trauma results in primary and secondary pathology. Primary pathology is injury to the brain tissue as a result of axonal and microcirculatory injury. This may result in cerebral edema (local or diffuse). Secondary pathology is injury to brain tissue as a result of damage to bridging veins, arteries, and dural sinuses. Primary pathology results in nonoperative lesions and management is limited to supportive care. Secondary pathology results in operative lesions in which damage to the brain may be mitigated by evacuation of hematomas through a hole in the skull. Surgical interventions for head injury have a long history in medicine. The use of trephination (drilling a hole in the head to relieve pressure) dates back to 3000 BC (Tello 1913). Modern surgical techniques and neuroimaging have greatly improved the success of neurosurgical interventions. The goal of evaluation in the acute care setting is to identify the patients with moderate to severe traumatic brain injury and to identify secondary pathology that can be addressed with a neurosurgical intervention.

6.3 Urgent Evaluation

After an immediate post injury assessment, the decision should be made whether or not the patient needs further medical evaluation. This decision is based on expert opinion and common sense. Most experts agree that there are red flags that suggest the possibility of more significant injury and the potential for progressive neurologic decline. Immediate symptoms, such as prolonged loss of consciousness (LOC) (more than a few seconds), seizures, neck pain, and focal neurologic signs (weakness, numbness, persistent visual disturbance), should prompt a referral to the ED to immediately exclude focal lesions that may require surgical intervention. For other patients, the persistence of severe symptoms such as worsening headache, repeated vomiting, behavior change, drowsiness, confusion, irritability, and/or slurred speech should prompt referral to the ED.

6.4 ED Evaluation

In the ED, the primary goals of TBI management are stabilizing the patient and identifying patients with significant or dynamic intracranial injuries. TBI is classified as mild, moderate, or severe based on acute injury characteristics. The most commonly used scale is the Glascow Coma Scale (GCS), which rates patient in eye opening (up to 4 points), verbal response (up to 5 points), and motor response (up to 6) on a scale from 3 to 15. Patients with GCS scores between 13 and 15 are deemed mild injuries, scores between 8 and 12 are classified as moderate, and scores less than 8 are considered severe. Patients who are classified as having a moderate/severe injury have a higher rate of clinically significant intracranial injury. While GCS is helpful in clinically distinguishing mild from moderate–severe TBI, there is a ceiling effect for mild TBI. While the majority of mild TBI patients are safe to discharge home, GCS does not account for severity or persistence of postconcussive symptoms. However, given that the primary focus of the ED evaluation is to identify the small subset of patients that need urgent neurosurgical intervention, GCS is a useful screening tool in this setting.

Of particular challenge in the ED is the evaluation of the mild TBI patients who have a small but nonzero rate of clinically significant intracranial injury. Research on clinical decision-making has thus been geared toward reducing the potential mortality of mTBI in these situations. There are few tools for use to evaluate injury severity in the ED setting other than observation and neuroimaging. In the pediatric population, it is rare to find clinically significant injury after 24 hours. Generally clinically significant injuries will present (with persistence or worsening of symptoms) within the first 4–8 hours after injury. In the ED setting, observing a patient for this long may not be practical and may delay treatment of surgical lesions. Neuroimaging has greatly improved outcomes following head trauma by allowing us to institute surgical intervention earlier. The most common imaging technique is CT scan. It is rapid, readily available, and can reliably detect clinically significant injuries. Potential drawbacks include possible need for transport out of the ED, pharmacologic sedation, and increase in the cost of care. Of additional increasing theoretical concern is the risk of lethal malignancy secondary to diagnostic radiation particularly in pediatric patients.

Over the past decade most studies of mTBI in the ED setting have focused on guidelines for neuroimaging (Atabaki et al. 2008; Haydel and Shembekar 2003; Palchak et al. 2003). The guidelines for the management of mTBI published in 1999 by the American Academy of Pediatrics focus primarily on an algorithm for detecting intracranial injury in acutely injured children (within 24 hours of injury) who have experienced a LOC of less than 1 minute (Bergman et al. 1999). While considered by many practitioners to be a cardinal sign of mTBI, LOC occurs in less than one quarter of individuals with mTBI (Collins et al. 2003; Schultz 2004). As a result, the AAP practice parameter concerns only a small percentage of children with mTBI and does not address the larger percentage group of children with mTBI without known LOC or intracranial injury.

Recently the Pediatric Emergency Care Applied Research Network conducted a large prospective cohort study of children <18 year old with mTBI (initial GCS of 14–15) to determine low risk criteria (Kuppermann et al. 2009). Subjects were assessed for clinically important TBI defined as neurosurgery, intubation, or hospitalization greater than 2 days. Over 42,000 patients were recruited over 2.4 years (33,785 to derive rule and 8,627 to validate). Only 376 (0.9%) had clinically important TBI. The study found that patients >2 years old are at extremely low risk for clinically important TBI if they have normal mental status, benign mechanism, no LOC, no vomiting, no severe headache, and no concern for basilar skull fracture. Application of this and other evidence into imaging guidelines could reduce unnecessary CT scans by 20%.

After the patient is stabilized and significant or dynamic intracranial injuries have been excluded, the clinician can shift focus to symptom management. The majority of symptoms can be managed by rest and observation. Many patients become very fatigued and sleepy following a head injury. The old adage that concussed patients should be kept awake was developed at a time when neuroimaging was not available. In the past, an acute change in level of consciousness may have been the only signal that a patient needed a neurosurgical intervention. With the advent of cranial CT, keeping patients awake is no longer necessary. In fact, sleep and rest may be the most effective ways to allow the brain to recover from concussion. While patients should be allowed to rest, they may be checked periodically (no more frequently than once an hour) to assess that they are easy to wake up and are acting appropriately.

Headache and nausea/vomiting are two common symptoms that are addressed in the acute care setting. Headache is usually migranous in nature (associated with photo/phono-phobia and nausea, improving with rest and sleep). Management of headache depends on severity. For mild to moderate symptoms, NSAIDs are the treatment of choice (7.5–10.0 mg/kg/dose). Acetaminophen (15 mg/kg/dose) is an appropriate though less effective alternative. Both of these medications have a low side effect profile. Triptans have been efficacious for adolescent migraine and are thought to act by constricting blood vessels and decreasing the release of inflammatory proteins. However, triptans have not been studied in the immediate postinjury setting and are not currently recommended.

For moderate to severe symptoms, more aggressive migraine treatment (such as IV fluids, prochlorperazine, or metoclopramide) may be initiated. Intravenous fluids with isotonic fluids (e.g., normal saline or lactated ringers) are a safe treatment method, though have not been studied as a stand-alone treatment. Prochlorperazine is a dopamine (D2) receptor antagonist that is used to treat nausea, dizziness (vertigo), and migraine headache. It is administered at 0.15 mg/kg with a maximum dose of 10 mg. The side effects are uncommon but include dyskinesia (e.g., dystonic reactions or akathesia), seizures, and has rarely been associated with neuroleptic malignant syndrome. Metoclopramide (0.1 mg/kg; maximum of 10 mg) acts as a D2 receptor antagonist with similar action and side effect profile but less efficacy. Opiate medications (e.g., morphine, oxycodone, hydrocodone, fentanyl) may be used, but are generally not recommended given the sedation associated with treatment and the lack of long-term efficacy.

Nausea and vomiting are common postconcussive complaints. For mild symptoms, oral ondansetron may be given. Ondansetron is a serotonin 5-HT_3 receptor antagonist which acts peripherally and centrally to decrease nausea. It has a very good safety profile. Patients who receive oral antiemetics should be observed for resolution of emesis. More significant symptoms may be addressed with IV therapy (e.g., ondansetron, prochlorperazine or metoclopramide) and IV fluids.

6.4.1   Admission

Some patients with mild traumatic brain injuries will require admission for observation, pain control, and/or hydration. Should more aggressive therapy for either headache or nausea (e.g., IV medications) be indicated, the provider should consider imaging to exclude significant intracranial injury.

Most patients with concussion will be able to be discharged home. Admission for observation should be considered in patients with persistent severe headache or emesis despite adequate therapy.

6.4.2   Outpatient Management

The actual course of symptom recovery is difficult to predict in the early stages while the neurometabolic cascade of brain injury is actively unfolding. The ED's role in follow-up care is to facilitate the ongoing treatment process by providing initial education regarding the injury, and communicate the patient's condition to the primary care system where follow up can continue.

Discharge instructions should provide information about the common postconcussive symptoms and emphasize the importance of rest and adequate oral intake. Providing patients with an explanation of what symptoms to expect and for how long has been shown to decrease reported symptoms at 3 months (Ponsford et al. 2001). For more severe head injury, maintaining an adequate perfusion and blood sugar prevents secondary injury. Similarly, patients with mild injury should stay well hydrated and eat well (specifically avoiding prolonged fasting). Above all, patients should be strongly advised to restrict physical activity which places them at risk for subsequent concussion until symptoms have resolved. This includes both returning to athletics and recreational activities (e.g., biking, rock climbing, riding rollercoasters). The literature has reported that postinjury physical and cognitive activities can have both positive and negative effects on recovery from concussion (Poirier 2003). Majerske and colleagues published a retrospective study of patients treated at a concussion center that demonstrated the complex association between postconcussive activity level and outcome (Majerske et al. 2008). Using a five-point activity scale coded on chart review, the study found that both patients with the lowest and highest levels of activity postinjury did poorly on follow-up neurocognitive testing using Immediate Postconcussion Assessment and Cognitive Testing (ImPACT). Patients with moderate levels of postinjury activity had better average scores at follow-up. In their discussion, the authors suggested that patients with lower activity levels had lower neurocognitive scores because they had more severe concussions to begin with. In contrast, they felt that patients with the highest activity levels overexerted themselves postinjury, thus worsening their outcomes.

The animal data on concussion suggests that timing of activity may explain the differences in outcome better than level of activity postinjury. One animal study of concussion found that concussed adult rats who were allowed physical activity in the first week postinjury performed poorly on follow-up neurocognitive tasks and had lower levels of a biochemical marker of neuron recovery. However, concussed rats who were allowed to exercise 2 weeks postinjury had improved performance and higher levels of recovery biomarkers (Griesbach et al. 2004). As for cognitive activity, animal studies of adult concussed rats have shown that a cognitively stimulating environment postinjury improved neurobehavioral outcomes (Maegele et al. 2005). However, in pediatric rat models, juvenile rats in the enriched environment showed greater neurobehavioral improvement if the stimulating environment was not introduced immediately following injury, but 2 weeks later (Giza et al. 2005). The plasticity of the juvenile brain may promote a tendency to create and maintain aberrant synaptic connections (Giza and Prins 2006). To date, there are no published human studies that have closely examined the relationship between the timing of cognitive activity and physical activity and recovery from concussion. Patients who are at high risk for subsequent concussion (athletes) or those who are at high risk for prolonged recovery (e.g., history of previous concussion or migraines) should be referred to a concussion specialist for follow up.

6.5 Summary

The goal of management during the early postinjury period is to stabilize the patient, exclude serious intracranial pathology, and guide recovery by encouraging rest and reduced metabolic activity. History and exam findings are used to determine if patients require emergent neuroimaging. Early symptoms are best managed with rest. Headache and nausea/vomiting may be managed medically. Above all the patient must receive adequate discharge education to ensure a safe recovery.

6.6   Key Points

Urgent evaluation is recommended for patients with certain immediate symptoms (such as prolonged LOC, seizures, neck pain, and focal neurologic signs) or persistent severe symptoms (such as worsening headache, repeated vomiting, behavior change, persistent drowsy appearance, increased confusion or irritability, and slurred speech).

Children with minor head injury are at extremely low risk for clinically important TBI and may be managed without emergent neuroimaging if they have normal mental status, benign mechanism, no LOC, no vomiting, no severe headache, and no concern for basilar skull fracture.

Rest and sleep should be encouraged following head injury.

Headache and nausea are common post concussive symptoms and may be managed with medications.

Discharge instructions should provide information about the common postconcussive symptoms and emphasize the importance of rest and avoidance of physical activities, which increase risk for subsequent concussion until symptoms have fully resolved.

References

(AAN), A. A. o. N. (1997). Practice parameter: the management of concussion in sports (summary statement). *Neurology, 48*, 581–585.

Atabaki, S. M., Stiell, I. G., Bazarian, J. J., Sadow, K. E., Vu, T. T., Camarca, M. A., et al. (2008). A clinical decision rule for cranial computed tomography in minor pediatric head trauma. *Archives of Pediatrics and Adolescent Medicine, 162*(5), 439–445.

Bergman, D. A., Baltz, R. D., Cooley, J. R., Coombs, J. B., Goldberg, M. J., Homer, C. J., et al. (1999). The management of minor closed head injury in children. *Pediatrics, 104*(6), 1407–1415.

CDC. (2007). *Heads up: brain injury in your practice.* Atlanta, GA: CDC.

Collins, M. W., Iverson, G. L., Lovell, M. R., McKeag, D. B., Norwig, J., & Maroon, J. (2003). On-field predictors of neuropsychological and symptom deficit following sports-related concussion. *Clinical Journal of Sports Medicine, 13*(4), 222–229.

Giza, C. C., Griesbach, G. S., & Hovda, D. A. (2005). Experience-dependent behavioral plasticity is disturbed following traumatic injury to the immature brain. *Behavioural Brain Research, 157*(1), 11–22.

Giza, C. C., & Prins, M. L. (2006). Is being plastic fantastic? Mechanisms of altered plasticity after developmental traumatic brain injury. *Developmental Neuroscience, 28*(4–5), 364–379.

Griesbach, G. S., Hovda, D. A., Molteni, R., Wu, A., & Gomez-Pinilla, F. (2004). Voluntary exercise following traumatic brain injury: brain-derived neurotrophic factor upregulation and recovery of function. *Neuroscience, 125*(1), 129–139.

Haydel, M. J., & Shembekar, A. D. (2003). Prediction of intracranial injury in children aged five years and older with loss of consciousness after minor head injury due to nontrivial mechanisms. *Annals of Emergency Medicine, 42*(4), 507–514.

Kuppermann, N., Holmes, J. F., Dayan, P. S., Hoyle, J. D., Jr., Atabaki, S. M., Holubkov, R., et al. (2009). Identification of children at very low risk of clinically-important brain injuries after head trauma: a prospective cohort study. *Lancet, 374*(9696), 1160–1170.

Langlois, J. A., Rutland-Brown, W., & Thomas, K. E. (2005). The incidence of traumatic brain injury among children in the United States: differences by race. *Journal of Head Trauma Rehabilitation, 20*(3), 229–238.

Maegele, M., Lippert-Gruener, M., Ester-Bode, T., Garbe, J., Bouillon, B., Neugebauer, E., et al. (2005). Multimodal early onset stimulation combined with enriched environment is associated with reduced CNS lesion volume and enhanced reversal of neuromotor dysfunction after traumatic brain injury in rats. *European Journal of Neuroscience, 21*(9), 2406–2418.

Majerske, C. W., Mihalik, J. P., Ren, D., Collins, M. W., Reddy, C. C., Lovell, M. R., et al. (2008). Concussion in sports: postconcussive activity levels, symptoms, and neurocognitive performance. *Journal of Athletic Training, 43*(3), 265–274.

Metzl, J. D. (2006). Concussion in the young athlete. *Pediatrics, 117*(5), 1813.

Palchak, M. J., Holmes, J. F., Vance, C. W., Gelber, R. E., Schauer, B. A., Harrison, M. J., et al. (2003). A decision rule for identifying children at low risk for brain injuries after blunt head trauma. *Annals of Emergency Medicine, 42*(4), 492–506.

Poirier, M. P. (2003). Concussions: assessment, management, and recommendations for return to activity. *Clinical Pediatric Emergency Medicine, 4*(3), 179–185.

Ponsford, J., Willmott, C., Rothwell, A., Cameron, P., Ayton, G., Nelms, R., et al. (2001). Impact of early intervention on outcome after mild traumatic brain injury in children. *Pediatrics, 108*(6), 1297–1303.

Schultz, M. (2004). Incidence and risk factors for concussion in high school athletes, North Carolina, 1996–1999. *American Journal of Epidemiology, 160*(10), 937–944.

Sosin, D. M., Sniezek, J. E., & Thurman, D. J. (1996). Incidence of mild and moderate brain injury in the United States, 1991. *Brain Injury, 10*(1), 47–54.

Tello, J. (1913). Pre-historic tephination among the Yamjos of Peru. 18th Session Congress Inter. des. Amer, pp. 75–83.

Chapter 7
Utilization of Imaging Technology in Concussion Assessment

Katherine S. Dahab and David T. Bernhardt

7.1 Introduction

The transient neurologic impairment resulting from a concussion is often frightening for parents and caretakers of the affected child. In the emergency room setting, children with concussions often undergo computed tomography (CT) scan to assess for structural damage in the brain. This "routine" use of imaging in children with concussion often adds little to the clinical management of the injury, as the vast majority of children with concussions have completely normal CT scans (McCrory et al. 2009). In addition, routine imaging with CT for the clinically uncomplicated concussion places children at risk for unnecessary radiation exposure. Although the imaging may reassure patients, families, and providers that no underlying severe structural injury is present, it does not predict the severity of concussion or guide postconcussion management.

Newer imaging techniques are more sensitive in the detection of the subtle, cellular-level changes associated with concussion. These newer techniques offer promise to help further reveal the true pathophysiology of concussions and may help better predict initial concussion severity and recovery. Most of the newer techniques are not yet well established with clinical use protocols but offer promise for the future.

K.S. Dahab (✉)
Primary Care Sports Medicine Fellow,
University of Wisconsin, Milwaukee, WI, USA
e-mail: katherine@thedahabs.com

D.T. Bernhardt
Department of Pediatrics, Orthopedics and Rehabilitation,
University of Wisconsin School of Medicine and Public Health,
Madison, WI, USA

J.N. Apps and K.D. Walter (eds.), *Pediatric and Adolescent Concussion:*
Diagnosis, Management and Outcomes, DOI 10.1007/978-0-387-89545-1_7,
© Springer Science+Business Media, LLC 2012

7.2 Computed Tomography

7.2.1 Technique and Indication

In the acute time period after injury (24–48 hours), CT scan is the imaging modality of choice to assess for structural intracranial injury, hemorrhage, or skull fracture (Miller et al. 1997; Hurley et al. 2004; Yealy and Hogan 1991). CT scans use a series of two-dimensional X-ray images, which are taken around a single axis of rotation to construct a 3D image of the brain (Fig. 7.1).

7.2.2 Recent Findings

A study published in 2010 sought to determine clinical criteria that could predict which patients are at high risk for intracranial injury after sustaining head trauma (Osmond et al. 2010). This study included primarily nonsport related concussions and all patients in this study did have a witnessed loss of consciousness (LOC).

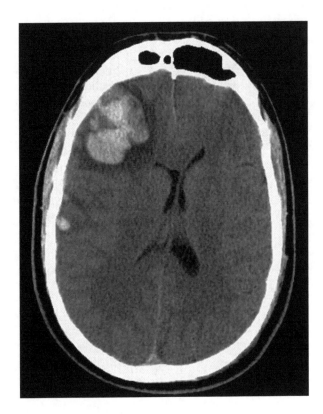

Fig. 7.1 Cranial CT Scan. Acute trauma CT showing hemorrhagic contusions in the right frontal lobe. Image courtesy of HA Rowley, MD

Clinical findings associated with structural brain injury in this study included a Glasgow Coma Score (GCS) of less than 15 at 2 hours after injury, suspected open or depressed skull fracture, history of worsening headache, and irritability on examination.

Reinforcing the above mentioned worrisome findings, other studies have also documented the clinical signs and symptoms that signal a more significant injury include loss of consciousness for more than thirty seconds, severe or worsening headaches, focal neurologic findings on exam, seizures, change in mental status, significant lethargy, slurred speech, repeated emesis, or neck pain. In addition, any child with progressively worsening symptoms after injury should be evaluated with neuroimaging to rule out a cervical spine injury, skull fracture, or intracranial hemorrhage (Fung et al. 2006). Children with a concussion but none of the above mentioned clinical findings are unlikely to have any abnormalities on CT imaging (Committee on Quality Improvement 1999).

7.2.3 Current Status

CT imaging will remain the imaging modality of choice in the acute setting to detect structural intracranial abnormalities and skull fractures when the clinical signs and symptoms are suspicious for a structural injury. In the setting of a concussion without any other worrisome clinical findings, CT scans do not have much utility. CT scans are of little use in the research setting because of the inability to detect subtle lesions of the brain.

7.3 Magnetic Resonance Imaging

7.3.1 Technique and Indication

Magnetic resonance imaging (MRI) is more sensitive than CT for detecting anatomical changes. MRI has higher resolution, the ability to image different planes and provide distinction between tissue types including gray matter, white matter, and cerebrospinal fluid. MRI uses a powerful magnetic field to align the magnetization of atoms in the brain. Once aligned, the MRI systematically changes the alignment of the magnetization via radio frequency fields. The resultant rotating magnetic fields produced by shifting nuclei are detectable by the scanner and are used to construct an image of the brain.

MRI is the test of choice if imaging is needed more than 48 hours after an injury. As mentioned above, worsening clinical symptoms would be the primary reason to pursue neuroimaging with suspicion for intracranial injury at that point (Fig. 7.2).

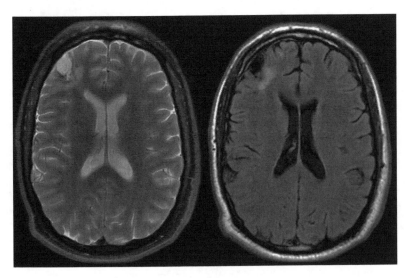

Fig. 7.2 Magnetic Resonance Imaging (MRI). MRI of the head shows evidence for focal cystic encephalomalcia at the site of prior contusion. The T2 images show dark stain at the margins indicative of hemosiderin from prior blood products. The T2 FLAIR images show surrounding high signal indicative of posttraumatic gliosis. Images courtesy of HA Rowley, MD

7.3.2   Recent Findings

MRI enables the detection of lesions such as cerebral contusion, petechial hemorrhage and white matter injury that can be missed on CT (Lee and Newberg 2005). Toga and Mazziotta demonstrated that the typical injuries detected by MRI after a sports-related concussion include small cortical contusions, subdural hematomas and small white matter hemorrhages. These injuries are thought to represent diffuse axonal injury in the brain (Toga and Mazziotta 2002).

7.3.3   Current Status

Though MRI provides enhanced resolution compared to CT, it is still not able to detect lesions in all concussed patients (Bazarian et al. 2006). MRI will remain the imaging modality of choice for concussed patients who are clinically worsening greater than 48 hours postinjury, but has little role in the management of otherwise uncomplicated concussions. Similar to CT scans, conventional MRI is not the focus of recent concussion research due to the inability to detect subtle lesions in the brain.

7.4   Diffusion Tensor Imaging

7.4.1   Technique and Indication

Diffusion tensor imaging (DTI) is a specific MRI technique that can detect axonal injury (Toga and Mazziotta 2002). This technique uses the differences of the restricted diffusion of water through gray and white matter in the brain to essentially map neural tracts and the direction in which they travel. In normal, healthy brains, the water molecules diffuse in an organized pattern. This directional organization is called anisotropy. In injured white matter, these neural tracks are less organized and this lack of organization, which indicates axonal injury, is detected by DTI (Fig. 7.3).

7.4.2   Recent Findings

The literature suggests a correlation between the severity of traumatic brain injury based on presenting GCS with the amount of diffuse axonal injury present on DTI (Huisman et al. 2004). There is a paucity of research in the literature focusing on acute concussion findings on DTI, especially in children. A few studies have demonstrated diffuse axonal injury in concussed patients using DTI within the first week of injury (Miles et al. 2008). In addition, one study showed a strong correlation between abnormal findings on DTI and clinical concussion symptoms (Wilde et al. 2008).

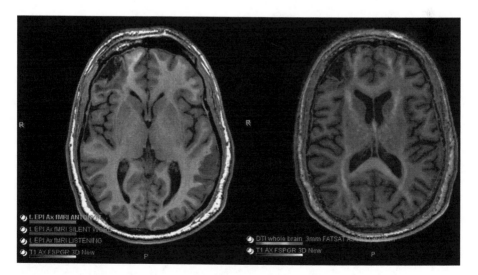

Fig. 7.3 Diffusion Tensor Imaging (DTI). Functional MRI (*left*) and diffusion tensor imaging (*right*) show intact left hemisphere language function but locally disturbed white matter connections related to the remote injury site. Images courtesy of HA Rowley, MD

7.4.3 Current Status

DTI holds promise for detecting axonal injury, which is thought to be one of the primary pathologies of concussion. More research is needed focusing on how DTI findings during the acute phase of concussion will help with clinical management and recovery curves.

7.5 Functional MRI

7.5.1 Technique and Indication

Functional imaging gives a glimpse of the cellular activity within the injured brain and enables measurement of metabolic and hemodynamic changes (Munson et al. 2006). Functional MRI (fMRI) was developed in the 1990s and utilizes the magnetic differences between oxygenated and deoxygenated hemoglobin to map hemodynamic changes related to neuronal activity. Oxygenated hemoglobin (oxyhemoglobin) is diamagnetic while deoxygenated hemoglobin (deoxyhemoglobin) is paramagnetic. Determining the subtle difference between the resultant MR signals is known as detecting the blood oxygen level dependent (BOLD) signal. Decreased blood flow to injured areas of the brain seen in such imaging is thought to represent a decreased functional capacity of the injured tissue.

7.5.2 Recent Findings

McAllister and colleagues demonstrated a correlation between concussion symptoms and changes in functional brain activation noted on fMRI (McAllister et al. 1999, 2001a, b). A few authors focused specifically on fMRI findings in concussed athletes. These studies, though small in number, suggested that athletes who had evidence of atypical or increased activation in the brain during a cognitive task on fMRI in the acute period after injury had longer recovery times than those with normal activation acutely after injury (Chen et al. 2004, 2007; Lovell et al. 2007). Chen and colleagues also demonstrated that concussed athletes with working memory problems had fMRIs with decreased signal in the dorsolateral prefrontal cortex. In addition, the degree of symptoms reported by concussed athletes corresponded with the degree of atypical BOLD signal on fMRI.

7.5.3   Current Status

Functional MRI also holds promise for advancing our understanding of neuropatho-logical changes that occur with concussion. More research is needed, especially in the pediatric population, to determine if certain findings on fMRI can help predict recovery time and concussion severity. These findings could also prove helpful for return to play decisions for young athletes. Further research and more availability of this imaging technique will be necessary before it can be recommended as a stan-dard technique for concussion assessment.

7.6   Positron Emission Tomography

7.6.1   Technique and Indication

Positron emission tomography (PET) uses emissions from intravenously injected radionuclides to construct exquisitely sensitive functional three-dimensional images of the brain. The injected radionuclide, which has a short half-life, is able to cross the blood–brain barrier and is distributed throughout the brain. Once injected, the patient is imaged in the PET scanner, which can detect blood flow, glucose and oxygen metabolism in brain tissues based on the radionuclide emissions.

7.6.2   Recent Findings

The majority of literature focusing on PET use in brain injury involves patients with severe brain injury. A few studies have looked at PET for more mild brain injury. Chen and colleagues evaluated the PET changes between five patients with persis-tent postconcussive symptoms after mild head trauma and five matched controls. Baseline resting PET imaging was similar in both groups. PET imaging performed while the subjects were performing a spatial working memory task, however, showed a difference in regional cerebral blood flow in the right prefrontal cortex in the injured group compared to the controls (Chen et al. 2003). This study suggested that injured brain tissues may only be detectable if imaged during a cognitive chal-lenge and may appear "normal" on PET imaging at rest. Gross and colleagues stud-ied 20 patients with more long-standing postconcussive symptoms. These patients, on average, had symptoms 43 months after injury. This study demonstrated an asso-ciation between metabolic abnormalities on PET imaging and neuropsychological assessments (Gross et al. 1996).

7.6.3   Current Status

PET imaging thus far demonstrates the ability to visualize metabolic disturbances during cognitive efforts in patients who have normal imaging at rest after brain injury. More studies focusing on changes in the acute phase after concussion and focusing specifically on the pediatric concussion population are needed before broad generalizations and recommendations can be made about this imaging technique. The need for an injected radioisotope makes this a more difficult technique to use in pediatric concussion research.

7.7   Single Photon Emission Computed Tomography

7.7.1   Technique and Indication

Single photon emission computed tomography (SPECT) is a technique similar to PET that enables visualization and assessment of cerebral perfusion after concussion. SPECT also requires an intravenous injection of a radioactive ligand, which crosses the blood–brain barrier and is distributed throughout the brain. Areas of brain tissue that require increased blood flow and nutrient delivery will accumulate higher amounts of the radioactive ligand and thus help construct a picture of regional cerebral blood flow.

7.7.2   Recent Findings

Most SPECT studies, similar to PET studies, focus on patients with persistent concussion symptoms stemming from a variety of initial injury mechanisms and do not focus on patients with concussions alone. Most of these studies demonstrate focal hypoperfusion in thalamic-basal ganglion areas and in frontal and temporal cortical areas on SPECT imaging (Abdel-Dayem et al. 1998; Abu-Judeh et al. 1999).

7.7.3   Current Status

Similar to PET imaging, more research focusing on acute changes associated with concussion is needed before the value of SPECT imaging for concussion management can be determined. The need for an injected radionuclide also makes this technique less attractive for research involving the pediatric concussion population.

7.8   Magnetic Resonance Spectroscopy

7.8.1   Technique and Indication

Magnetic resonance spectroscopy (MRS) is a noninvasive imaging technique that enables the detection of neuronal damage and neurochemical changes after brain injury (Babikian et al. 2006; Belanger et al. 2005). MRS measures specific metabolites within the brain including N-acetylaspartate (NAA), which is a marker of neuronal integrity; myoinositol, a glial marker; creatine, a general energy marker; choline, a marker of membrane turnover and neuronal injury; and lactate, which is an indirect marker of ischemia.

7.8.2   Recent Findings

MRS imaging has shown changes in ratios of these markers in patients who have mild brain injury compared to control populations, even when no detectable abnormalities are found on conventional MRI. Furthermore, MRS studies suggest that this technique can identify metabolic derangements in brain tissue after injury even when clinical symptoms have resolved (Vagnozzi et al. 2008).

7.8.3   Current Status

MRS holds promise for helping to guide return to play decision-making for young athletes since it can identify lingering metabolic abnormalities within the brain after injury even when patients report resolution of clinical symptoms. More research is needed to determine the extent to which this imaging can help with concussion management.

7.9   Summary of Research Findings

Conventional neuroimaging such as CT and MRI are useful if the clinical picture suggests possible intracranial injury in addition to the concussion, but has little use in concussion management. CT and MRI are not sensitive enough to detect the subtle brain injury. Functional imaging modalities such as fMRI, PET, SPECT and MRS are able to detect the cellular level changes associated with mild traumatic brain injuries. Since there is no true "gold standard" of imaging for concussions, it is difficult to determine the sensitivity, specificity, positive or negative predictive value of any of these newer imaging modalities. More research and wider availability of these techniques is needed before more general recommendations can be made for their use in concussion management.

7.10   Key Points

Conventional imaging, such as CT and MRI, are often normal in concussion and often do not add much to the diagnostic or prognostic data.

Red flag signs and symptoms indicating the need for conventional neuroimaging include any worsening symptoms, loss of consciousness for more than thirty seconds, severe or worsening headaches, focal neurologic findings on exam, seizures, change in mental status, significant lethargy, slurred speech, repeated emesis, or neck pain.

CT scan is the imaging modality of choice to assess for intracranial injury or skull fracture acutely after an injury (within the first 24 hours).

MRI may be a more appropriate choice for patients with unusual worsening symptoms greater than 48 hours after injury.

Functional imaging enables the visualization of more subtle injury findings in concussion. Though promising, these techniques are not yet well established or recommended for routine use in concussion management.

Additional research is needed in all of these imaging modalities focusing on their diagnostic and prognostic capabilities during concussion management. None of the above mentioned techniques are yet recommended for routine use in concussion management.

References

Abdel-Dayem, H. M., Abu-Judeh, H., Kumar, H., et al. (1998). SPECT brain perfusion abnormalities in mild or moderate traumatic brain injury. *Clinical Nuclear Medicine, 23*, 309–317.

Abu-Judeh, H. H., Parker, R., Singh, M., et al. (1999). SPECT brain perfusion imaging in mild traumatic brain injury without loss of consciousness and normal computed tomography. *Nuclear Medicine Communications, 20*, 505–510.

Babikian, T., Freier, M. C., Ashwal, S., et al. (2006). MR spectroscopy: predicting long-term neuropsychological outcome following pediatric TBI. *Journal of Magnetic Resonance Imaging, 24*, 801–811.

Bazarian, J. J., Blythe, B., & Cimpello, L. (2006). Bench to bedside: evidence for brain injury after concussion – looking beyond the computed tomography scan. *Academic Emergency Medicine, 13*(2), 199–214.

Belanger, H. G., Curtiss, G., Demery, J. A., et al. (2005). Factors moderating neuropsychological outcomes following mild traumatic brain injury: a meta-analysis. *Journal of International Neuropsychological Society, 11*, 215–227.

Chen, J. K., Johnston, K. M., Collie, A., McCrory, P., & Ptito, A. (2007). A validation of the post concussion symptom scale in the assessment of complex concussion using cognitive testing and functional MRI. *Journal of Neurology, Neurosurgery, and Psychiatry, 78*, 1231–1238.

Chen, J. K., Johnston, K. M., Frey, S., et al. (2004). Functional abnormalities in symptomatic concussed athletes: an fMRI study. *NeuroImage, 22*, 68–82.

Chen, S. H., Kareken, D. A., Fastenau, P. S., et al. (2003). A study of persistent post-concussion symptoms in mild head trauma using positron emission tomography. *Journal of Neurology, Neurosurgery, and Psychiatry, 74*, 326–332.

Committee on Quality Improvement, American Academy of Pediatrics, Commission of Clinical Policies and Research, American Academy of Family Physicians. (1999). The management of minor closed head injury in children. *Pediatrics, 104*, 1407–1415.

Fung, M., Willer, B., Moreland, D., & Leddy, J. (2006). A proposal for an evidence-based emergency department discharge form for mild traumatic brain injury. *Brain Injury, 20*(9), 889–94.

Gross, H., Kling, A., Henry, G., Herndon, C., & Lavretsky, H. (1996). Local cerebral glucose metabolism in patients with long-term behavioral and cognitive deficits following mild traumatic brain injury. *The Journal of Neuropsychiatry and Clinical Neurosciences, 8*, 324–334.

Huisman, T. A., Schwamm, L. H., Schaefer, P. W., et al. (2004). Diffusion tensor imaging as potential biomarker of white matter injury in diffuse axonal injury. *American Journal of Neuroradiology, 25*, 370–376.

Hurley, R. A., McGowan, J. C., Arfanakis, K., & Taber, K. H. (2004). Traumatic axonal injury: novel insights into evolution and identification. *The Journal of Neuropsychiatry and Clinical Neurosciences, 16*(1), 1–7.

Lee, B., & Newberg, A. (2005). Neuroimaging in traumatic brain imaging. *NeuroRx, 2*(2), 372–383.

Lovell, M. R., Pardini, J. E., Welling, J., et al. (2007). Functional brain abnormalities are related to clinical recovery and time to return to play in athletes. *Neurosurgery, 61*, 352–359.

McAllister, T. W., Saykin, A. J., Flashman, L. A., et al. (1999). Brain activation during working memory 1 month after mild traumatic brain injury: a functional MRI study. *Neurology, 53*, 1300–1308.

McAllister, T. W., Sparling, M. B., Flashman, L. A., et al. (2001a). Differential working memory load effects after mild traumatic brain injury. *NeuroImage, 14*, 1004–1012.

McAllister, T. W., Sparling, M. B., Flashman, L. A., et al. (2001b). Neuroimaging findings in mild traumatic brain injury. *Journal of Clinical and Experimental Neuropsychology, 23*, 775–791.

McCrory, P., Meeuwisse, W., Johnston, K., et al. (2009). Consensus statement on Concussion in Sport 3rd International Conference on Concussion in Sport held in Zurich, November 2008. *Clinical Journal of Sport Medicine, 19*(3), 185–200.

Miles, L., Grossman, R. I., Johnsoh, G., et al. (2008). Short-term DTI predictors of cognitive dysfunction in mild traumatic brain injury. *Brain Injury, 22*, 115–122.

Miller, E. C., Holmes, J. F., & Derlet, R. W. (1997). Utilizing clinical factors to reduce head CT scan ordering for minor head trauma patients. *The Journal of Emergency Medicine, 15*(4), 453–457.

Munson, S., Schroth, E., & Ernst, M. (2006). The role of functional neuroimaging in pediatric brain injury. *Pediatrics, 117*, 1372–1381.

Osmond, M. H., Klassen, T. P., Wells, G. A., et al. (2010). CATCH: a clinical decision rule for the use of computerized tomography in children with minor head injury. *Canadian Medical Association Journal, 182*(4), 1372–1381.

Toga, A. W., & Mazziotta, J. C. (2002). *Brain mapping: the methods* (2nd ed.). San Diego, CA: Academic.

Vagnozzi, R., Signoretti, S., Tavazzi, B., et al. (2008). Temporal window of metabolic brain vulnerability to concussion: a pilot 1 H-magnetic resonance spectroscopic study in concussed athletes – part III. *Neurosurgery, 62*, 1286–1295.

Wilde, E. A., McCauley, S. R., Hunter, J. V., et al. (2008). Diffusion tensor imaging of acute mild traumatic brain injury in adolescents. *Neurology, 70*, 948–955.

Yealy, D. M., & Hogan, D. E. (1991). Imaging after head trauma: who needs what? *Emergency Medicine Clinics of North America, 9*(4), 707–717.

Chapter 8
Long-Term Assessment of Concussion

Jonathan E. Romain

8.1 Introduction

Few topics in medicine inspire more debate among professionals than the long-term consequences of concussion. A major reason for this is the vast majority of patients sustaining mild traumatic brain injury (mTBI) have full and complete recovery, returning to normal activities often within days of the injury (Carroll et al. 2004). However, a subset of individuals will have symptoms persisting for weeks to months, and even years. These persisting and often elusive symptoms can be difficult to manage and can cause a great deal of frustration for patients and their families, as well as the clinicians hoping to alleviate them. Protracted recovery is generally divided into two categories, with a fair bit of overlap. Symptoms lasting beyond a few days to greater than a week represent postconcussion syndrome (PCS). Depending on how it is defined, PCS is felt to occur in up to 20% of concussion patients, though more recent literature estimates the prevalence rate to be less than 5% (Iverson 2005). An even smaller group of patients will have symptoms persisting well beyond the duration of the typical recovery process, leading to what has been termed persistent postconcussion syndrome (PPCS) (Alexander 1995). As currently defined, PPCS represents symptoms lasting greater than 3 months (Bigler 2008). What we do know from the extant research is that symptom recovery varies by injury severity, and generally children tend to have a more protracted recovery course with more apparent cognitive changes following a concussion, making PCS and PPCS an essential topic for discussion in this book (Field et al 2003). Within the pediatric setting, there also exists a group of patients who have devastating consequences following an otherwise minor head injury, where a cascade of diffuse cerebral swelling and edema results in severe deficits or death (McCrory 2001), though this is not discussed here.

J.E. Romain (✉)
Department of Psychiatry and Behavioral Medicine,
Children's Hospital of Wisconsin, Milwaukee, WI, USA
e-mail: Jromain@chw.org

J.N. Apps and K.D. Walter (eds.), *Pediatric and Adolescent Concussion:*   93
Diagnosis, Management and Outcomes, DOI 10.1007/978-0-387-89545-1_8,
© Springer Science+Business Media, LLC 2012

Many children and adolescents in clinical practice are referred for assessment of cognitive and emotional/behavioral symptoms in the context of a relatively recent but occasionally remote concussion. These patients are often complex, presenting with multiple layers of elusive symptoms recalcitrant to well-designed and orchestrated rest and recovery plans, and accommodations and supports in the classroom. Treating providers are frustrated by the inability to relieve symptoms, schools do not know how to get the child back "on track," parents do not know what else to do for their child, and patients are left frustrated and at times resolved to the perception that he/she is inexorably head injured. Clearly, the impact of concussion extends far beyond the initial injury.

The aim of this chapter is to review the history of and current research on the persistent symptoms of concussion. It is hoped that a clearer understanding of the symptoms of PCS and PPCS will help the reader to have a better handle on the second goal of this chapter, which is to identify the utility and limitations of assessment tools in identifying and managing persistent concussion. Significant variation exists in the clinical management of concussion, and the continued development of assessment and management tools will be instrumental in gaining consensus in pediatric concussion management. A discussion of the controversies in the literature regarding definitions and diagnostic criteria is inevitable, but is kept to a minimum except as it relates to the need for further research.

8.2 Discussion of Relevant Terms and Review of Current Research

8.2.1 Postconcussion Syndrome

As stated, PCS refers to the presence of symptoms persisting typically days to a few weeks beyond the initial injury. While again noted here that the vast majority of patients with concussion will return to baseline functioning within hours to days, recovery varies as a function of injury characteristics (e.g., complicated vs. uncomplicated), as well as individual and demographic variables. For example, we know from moderate and severe traumatic brain injury (TBI) that earlier age at time of injury, history of preexisting learning difficulties, and premorbid psychiatric issues all contribute to the overall prognosis. The same appears to hold true for concussion. We also tend to see presence of life stressors at the time of injury and the resulting intensification of those stressors (due to days missed from school, sports, and/or activities) as a major factor in symptom reports, especially with adolescents.

In general, PCS symptoms can be categorized in terms of somatic, cognitive, and emotional sequelae occurring with varying frequency depending on the study (Mittenberg et al. 1997), with cognitive and somatic symptoms occurring with greatest frequency in children (Ayr et al. 2009). These authors noted that, while behavioral issues are observed in children during the early phase of concussion, they are not consistently seen in children with PCS. It is important to recognize here that symptoms often overlap within and between categories such that a somatic symptom (e.g., headache) can contribute to attention or memory problems (i.e., a cognitive complaint), and also can exacerbate or even precipitate an emotional or behavioral expression (e.g., depression or irritability). Further compounding the situation is these symptoms are common to other disorders potentially associated with concussion (e.g., posttraumatic stress disorder, chronic pain, etc.). However, perhaps the greatest issue in defining and identifying PCS is that various specialties use different sets of diagnostic criteria to diagnose the syndrome, which precludes generalizability across the research studies.

8.2.1.1 Somatic Symptoms

Headache and dizziness constitute the most common physical manifestation following a head injury and tend to be the most persistent, with headaches reported in upward of 70% of patients with PCS (Hall et al. 2005). Acute headaches are considered to largely resolve within the first 3 months of injury though between 8 and 32% of concussion patients still report headache 12 months after the injury. In 2009, Stovner et al. (2009) addressed headache and concussion concluding that, at least in adults, pretraumatic headache was a strong predictor of posttraumatic headache. It was also found that headache occurring 3 months or more after concussion may represent "primary headache" possibly as a function of stress rather than direct consequence of cerebral insult. It is, therefore, important to consider various factors contributing to postconcussion headache.

Dizziness tends to occur in adults and geriatric patients with greater frequency than children and may more typically reflect disturbance within the vestibular system. Other somatic symptoms include photo-and phonophobia, tinnitus, and blurred vision. The frequency of these symptoms within the pediatric population has not been fully established.

Problems with sleep are also common following concussion. Many children report excess need for sleep, while others report trouble falling asleep. These issues are seen with greater frequency when patients are restricted from school and extra-curricular activities for extended periods and are therefore off their typical routines. Anecdotally, many children coming through the author's clinic often confidentially report an increase in their television watching, videogame playing, and Internet browsing when restricted from school, despite doctor orders to avoid such activities, and much of this is occurring late into the evening when parents are not awake to monitor their child's behavior. Direct education with the patient regarding the strain to eyes and other senses caused by these seemingly "passive" activities may help curb excessive TV and Internet. It further appears that many sleep–wake cycle problems tend to resolve with cessation of late-night TV and Internet and upon more generally reestablishing a routine and resuming normal activity (i.e., return to school).

It is clear that somatic symptoms represent a significant area of concern in the management of PCS, particularly when considering improvement in somatic symptoms often has a cascade effect resulting in improved cognitive and emotional functioning.

That being said, there is evidence that cognitive symptoms tend to persist to some degree beyond the resolution of physical symptoms, which is discussed in more detail in the section that follows.

8.2.1.2 Cognitive

Cognitive issues occurring immediately after a concussion are common. As discussed in additional chapters, several tools exist to aid the clinician in the evaluation of concussion severity and symptoms immediately after and in the days following the injury. Symptoms of inattention, lack of focus, fogginess, decreased ability to keep information in mind to process (i.e., working memory), and memory disturbance are considered the hallmark of concussion. Cognitive symptoms tend to vary by injury severity, among other factors, and tend to resolve with time and appropriate concussion management.

Neuropsychological *evaluation* can be extremely helpful in addressing the complex interplay between cognitive, psychological, and somatic symptoms that exist with neurological disruption; however, neuropsychological *testing* itself is not used for the explicit purpose of diagnosing brain damage. The distinction here between evaluation and testing is an evaluation includes a comprehensive review of records and integration of several pieces of information regarding premorbid and current functioning, along with interpretation of test results, while neuropsychological testing is the administration of paper/pencil or computer based tasks and comparing an individual's performance to a normative sample. Without the context of background information, test scores in isolation cannot reliably distinguish brain-based deficits from, for example, deficits as a result of emotional disturbance (e.g., depression). Additionally, evidence among adults with PCS suggests that traditional neuropsychological measures lack sensitivity necessary for detecting impairment in concussion, particularly as it pertains to return to play determinations in sports medicine (Randolph et al. 2009). That said, deficits in neuropsychological functioning have been observed in the pediatric PCS population to suggest a degree of sensitivity to disturbance in brain function, particularly in the areas of sustained attention, processing speed and general reaction time, working memory, planning, and inhibition (Yeates et al. 1999; Iverson et al. 2006). Thus, it is not surprising that there is mixed support for the utility of neuropsychological *testing* in the diagnosis of PCS. A more detailed review of the use of neuropsychological measures in pediatric concussion is contained in other chapters of this text, though it is offered here that the complex interplay between somatic, emotional, and cognitive symptoms central to concussion warrants a comprehensive neuropsychological evaluation, which may or may not include extensive neuropsychological testing.

8.2.1.3 Emotional

The emotional toll following an injury is undeniable, particularly when the injury involves a child, and even more so when that child has sustained trauma involving the head. This perception of severity may relate to symptoms of disrupted consciousness or posttraumatic amnesia (PTA) (when present) that suggest to the patient and caregiver that a major injury has occurred. During a recent evaluation of a patient who had struck his head resulting in brief loss of consciousness (LOC) during a basketball game 6 months prior to his assessment, the child's mother remarked to the effect that her child's injury would not have been that concerning if it were not for the fact that he "hit his brain." She had read about concussion through some literature offered to parents and retained the message that a concussion is a serious injury.

It should not come as a surprise to the clinician that emotional reactions can result from an otherwise uncomplicated concussion. Combine this with the potential for somatic symptoms and cognitive complaints, and emotional difficulties are to be expected. Awareness and management of emotional issues (e.g., depression and anxiety) following an injury is further underlined by research demonstrating that cognitive improvements are often observed with treatment with psychotropics (Fann et al. 2001). The challenges in assessing and managing emotional and behavioral changes are further compounded by the fact that affective disturbance and increased emotional lability are often a direct consequence of neurologic disruption, particularly the prefrontal system.

8.2.2 Persistent Postconcussion Syndrome

The term Persistent Postconcussion Syndrome or PPCS was first coined by Alexander in 1995 to describe patients with milder brain injury (i.e., Glasgow Coma Scale (GCS) 13–15; LOC less than 10 min; PTA less than 1 hour) whose symptoms extend beyond 1 year. At that point, his research was suggesting approximately 15% of patients with concussion would be expected to exhibit debilitating symptoms at the 1 year postinjury mark. Since that time there has been some contention over the prevalence and even the very existence of PPCS as a neurophysiologic construct. Some consensus has been achieved in that most researchers and clinicians agree that a small percentage of individuals suffering a concussion will have symptoms extending beyond the typical recovery course; however, the mechanisms perpetuating these symptoms remain enthusiastically debated.

One fairly clear consensus is that premorbid neurological and psychiatric syndromes place individuals at greater risk for persistent symptoms following a concussion (Ponsford 2005), and this is consistent with our understanding that in more severe forms of TBI there tends to be a magnification of prior academic struggles and premorbid neuropsychiatric issues. However, evidence also supports exogenous factors (e.g., socioeconomic status, presence of life stressors) as placing individuals at greater risk for PPCS. There is further an undeniable body of literature showing that patients involved in litigation tend to have more persistent symptoms (Hall et al. 2005), and not surprisingly, this latter fact has the potential to weigh heavily on the minds of the treating providers working with concussion patients. Regardless of whether patients are litigious, clinicians need to remain objective and not make injudicious assumptions that PPCS reflects malingering or feigning of symptoms for secondary gain, monetary or otherwise.

One would expect that severity of the injury (keeping in mind that concussion theoretically represents the spectrum of mild head injury) would have some predictive value in identifying PPCS but this has not proven to be the case (Guskiewicz et al. 2004). It remains to be seen whether advances in neuroimaging (e.g., diffusion tensor MRI) will help to better link injury severity with residual impairment. In the meantime, clinicians need to bear in mind that persistent symptoms of pain, fatigue, changes in cognition, and mood disturbance are often overlapping. Thus, we need to be ever mindful of the many factors contributing to persistent postconcussion symptoms when evaluating our patients and providing appropriate treatment recommendations.

In summary, premorbid neurological and psychiatric syndromes place individuals at greater risk for persistent symptoms following a concussion, and this is consistent with our understanding that in more severe forms of TBI there tends to be a magnification of prior academic struggles and premorbid neuropsychiatric issues. Additionally, severity of the concussion does not appear to have predictive value in identifying PPCS. Lastly, there continues to be suspicion for a psychogenic component to PPCS, while research is continuing to explore the underlying neurophysiologic consequences of mild TBI to better understand why some individuals have lingering symptoms.

8.3   The Assessment of Persistent Concussion

The variable nature of concussion and rapidly changing post injury characteristics would suggest that monitoring the course of recovery over time might be of greater importance than appreciating the characteristics of the concussion at the time of injury. This particularly holds true when considering the aforementioned interplay between cognitive, somatic, and emotional symptoms observed in the context of protracted concussion. Additionally, the goals of assessment at different stages of concussion tend to change as the child progresses through the recovery process. This section focuses on some of the assessment tools currently used to evaluate children with PCS and PPCS, including an exploration of symptom-based measures, broad based behavior rating scales, and clinic-based cognitive performance tests. A more in-depth examination of neuropsychological and computer testing will be had in later chapters of this text.

One challenge, particularly for researchers attempting to advance our knowledge of mTBI, relates to inconsistencies among diagnostic criteria for PCS. For example, the two most commonly used diagnostic criteria for PCS, the *10th Edition of the International Classification of Diseases (ICD-10)* and the *Diagnostic and Statistical Manual of Mental Disorders -Fourth Edition- Text Revision (DSM-IV-TR)* (see Tables 8.1 and 8.2), vary regarding nomenclature.

Table 8.1 ICD-10 diagnostic criteria for postconcussional syndrome

A. History of head trauma with loss of consciousness precedes symptoms onset by maximum of 4 weeks
B. Symptoms in three or more of the following symptom categories:
   * Headache, dizziness, malaise, fatigue, noise tolerance
   * Irritability, depression, anxiety, emotional liability
   * Subjective concentration, memory, or intellectual difficulties without neuropsychological evidence or marked impairment
   * Insomnia
   * Reduced alcohol tolerance
   * Preoccupation with above symptoms and fear of brain damage with hypochondriacal concern and adoption of sick role

From International Statistical Classification of Diseases and Related Health Problems, 10th edn.

Table 8.2 DSM-IV research criteria for postconcussional disorder

A. A history of head trauma that has caused significant cerebral concussion. Note: The manifestations of concussion include loss of consciousness, posttraumatic amnesia, and, less, commonly, posttraumatic onset of seizures. The specific method of defining this criterion needs to be established be further research.
B. Evidence from neuropsychological testing or qualified cognitive assessment of difficulty in attention (concentrating, shifting focus of attention, performing simultaneous cognitive tasks) or memory (Learning or recall of information).
C. Three (or more) of the following occur shortly after the trauma and last at least 3 months:
   1. Becoming fatigued easily
   2. Disordered sleep
   3. Headache
   4. Vertigo or dizziness
   5. Irritability or aggression on little or no provocation
   6. Anxiety, depression, or affective instability
   7. Changes in personality (e.g., social or sexual inappropriateness)
   8. Apathy of lack of spontaneity
D. The symptoms in criteria B and C have their onset following head trauma or else represent a substantial worsening of preexisting problems.
E. The disturbance causes significant impairment in social or occupational functioning and represents a significant decline from a previous level of functioning. In school-age children, the impairment may be manifested by a single worsening in school or academic performance dating form the trauma.
F. The symptoms do not meet criteria for Dementia Due to Head Trauma and are not better accounted for by another mental disorder (e.g., Amnestic Disorder Due to Head Trauma, Personality Change Due to Head Trauma).

From Diagnostic and Statistical Manual of Mental Disorders, 4th edn.

As pointed out in previous works (McCrea 2008), both sets of criteria require an injury with resultant LOC despite that it has been documented for years that cognitive alteration (most often memory disturbance) can occur without positive LOC (Yarnell 1970; Ommaya and Gennarelli 1974). A study by Boake et al. (2005) revealed large discrepancies in the prevalence of PCS between the DSM-IV and ICD-10 to suggest that diagnosis using these criteria is not recommended without further refinement of the categories. Lack of consistency in the use of PCS criteria not only contributes to variability in sample ascertainment resulting in wide discrepancies between studies but underscores the need for sensitive and specific tools to better identify and diagnose PCS. Additionally, given the variability in injury severity and multiple dimensions contributing to outcome, along with the lack of consistency among specialties in developing a consensus diagnosis for PCS, it is essential to implement and further develop valid and reliable assessment tools to better assess for concussion so that we can then match treatment plans with the individual needs of the patient.

Assessment of the post acute phase of recovery in children with persistent concussion symptoms ideally requires the expertise and support of trainers, coaches, caregivers, and medical professionals all working in collaboration to understand the child's unique situation. Each of these providers can offer a distinct perspective to multiple dimensions across multiple settings (e.g., school, home, playing field), and it bears repeating that primary care providers (i.e., parents) should be actively involved in the assessment process throughout.

8.3.1 Symptom-Based Rating Scales

Various scales have been developed or adopted from adult concussion rating scales for the purpose of monitoring recovery. Some of these measures have shown strong psychometric properties necessary to assess postconcussion symptom severity, while others are in need of further refinement (Gioia et al. 2009). The Concussion Symptom Inventory (CSI) is a 27-item subjective symptom checklist that has been shown to be sensitive in the identification of concussion symptoms particularly in the sports-related setting (Randolph et al. 2009). Another scale that has been used with some interest in the pediatric population is the Concussion Symptom Checklist (Miller and Mittenberg 1998), which is a questionnaire that asks parents to report the presence or absence of 12 symptoms during the preceding week within the core domains of cognitive, somatic, and emotional functioning (see Table 8.3). The symptoms addressed by this scale also appear loosely based on both ICD and DSM criteria.

The Postconcussion Symptom Inventory (PCSI) is a 26-item, 7-point Likert scale that has more recently been modified for use with children, as well as parents and teachers, and emphasizes the physical, cognitive, and behavioral symptoms of concussion. This measure also assesses the sleep domain. The added benefit of this tool is that two forms exist to capture a retrospective preinjury level of functioning, which is then compared with a postinjury report of symptoms.

The Postconcussion Scale (PCS) is a self-report measure of severity of concussion symptoms and also allows for responses in a Likert scale format. These and similar scales provide a framework for structured interview, but caution should be exercised in using these tools in isolation (i.e., in the absence of gaining a thorough history), as they often provide only a snapshot of a multidimensional picture. Responses to questions on these types of symptom rating inventories must be taken in context with the child's age and developmental level, although, there appears to be a trend toward designing symptom inventories with age-specificity in mind.

Table 8.3 Concussion symptom checklist

1. Have you had *headaches* during the last week?	——
How many days were you bothered by these headaches during the last week?	——
How bad are the headaches usually, on a scale from 1 to 10?	——
2. Have you had *anxiety* during the past week?	——
How many days where you bothered by this anxiety during the last week?	——
How bad is the anxiety usually, on a scale from 1 to 10?	——
3. Have you had *depression* during the past week?	——
How many days where you bothered by this depression during the past week?	——
How bad is the depression usually, on a scale from 1 to 10?	——
4. Have you had *difficulty concentrating* during the last week?	——
How many days where you bothered by *concentration problems* during the last week?	——
How bad is your concentration, on a scale from 1 to 10?	——
5. Have you had any *dizziness* during the last week?	——
How many days where you bothered by dizziness during the last week?	——
How bad is the dizziness, on a scale from 1 to 10?	——
6. Have you had *trouble remembering things* during the past week?	——
How many days did you have trouble remembering things during the last week?	——
How bad are the memory problems, on a scale from 1 to 10?	——
7. Have you had *blurry or double vision* during the last week?	——
How many days were you bothered by vision problems during the last week?	——
How bad is the blurry or double vision usually, on a scale from 1 to 10?	——
8. Have you had *trouble thinking* during the past week?	——
How many days did you have trouble thinking or the last week?	——
How bad is the trouble thinking usually, on a scale from 1 to 10?	——
9. Have you been *irritable* during the past week?	——
How many days were you irritable during the last week?	——
How bad is the irritability usually, on a scale from 1 to 10?	——
10. Have you been *tired* a lot during the past week?	——
How many days were you tired a lot during the last week?	——
How tired have you been usually, on a scale from 1 to 10?	——
11. Have you been *sensitive to bright light* during the last week?	——
How many days were you light sensitive during the last week?	——
How bad is the sensitivity usually come on a scale from 1 to 10?	——
12. Have you been *sensitive to loud noise* during the last week?	——
How many days were you sensitive to loud noise during the last week?	——
How bad is the noise sensitivity usually, on a scale from 1 to 10?	——

Miller and Mittenberg (1998)

8.3.2 Behavior Rating Scales

Behavior rating scales have been used for decades with children for assessment of mood and behavior in the context of psychiatric and neuropsychiatric disorders. These measures typically provide an assessment of internalizing (acting in) and externalizing (acting out) behaviors, as well as attention and social functioning. Rating scales such as the Achenbach Child Behavior Checklist (CBCL) (Achenbach 1978) have been used for years with the broad TBI population and also appear to have utility in the assessment of the emotional well-being of the child with concussion.

As noted, understanding preinjury characteristics, such as developmental level, history of learning struggles and premorbid psychiatric and behavioral issues is crucial in understanding the context of symptoms and tailoring an appropriate treatment plan. This added dimension can shed much needed light on symptom checklists by helping clinicians determine symptoms that might be less likely a function of the actual concussion. For example, an endorsement of persistent concentration problems might be easier to interpret and manage if the child has a known prior history of anxiety. In this particular scenario, treatment might focus more on cognitive and behavioral strategies specifically geared toward anxiety reduction than on a cognitive remediation plan to help improve "concentration." One might assume that caregivers would make an obvious connection between premorbid functioning and current symptoms but this is not always the case. In some situations, preexisting symptoms are subsurface or subclinical, causing minimal apparent disturbance until they are amplified by a head injury, and only a more focused exploration of the child's earlier temperament, behavior, and general coping strategies before the injury can shed light on the contribution of such issues.

8.3.3 Standardized Testing

Formal cognitive assessment has been shown to be beneficial for children with persistent symptoms; however, the trend is moving toward employing more focused assessment of known head injury characteristics over an extensive neuropsychological battery of tests. In this author's multidisciplinary setting, where primarily moderate TBI patients are evaluated, a fairly fixed battery of tests is employed including selected "fluid reasoning" subtests from the Wechsler scales, a continuous performance measure looking at sustained attention and impulse control, a list learning task with delay and recognition components, a brief motor exam, and select executive function measures. Formal testing lasts approximately 90 min, and additional measures are added to the battery should further exploration be necessary. These test results are incorporated with information obtained from family on prior home and school functioning as well as current symptoms, and are used to develop an action plan. Computer testing will be discussed in other chapters but has undeniable benefit in efficiency of administration, also affording the opportunity to repeat measures in fairly rapid succession to closely monitor functioning over time. There is also the benefit of potentially having baseline testing, though, baseline testing has its own set of potential confounds. Additionally, as with all testing, consistent effort and motivation need to be controlled for to ensure meaningful test results. Testing with an examiner in a one:one environment tends to maximize the likelihood of obtaining valid results and observation of testing behaviors can further inform test results. Adult neuropsychologists have been using various symptom validity tests (SVTs) to assess for motivation and effort, and more recently these types of measures have been finding their way into the pediatric neuropsychology practice.

An additional dimension that needs to be addressed when managing children with PCS is assessment of parent response and adjustment to the injury, which literature suggests has a significant mitigating factor in the perpetuation of emotional and behavioral symptoms in children (Yeates and Taylor 2005). More specifically, level of parent anxiety has been shown to contribute to the severity and duration of PCS, as it relates to returning to daily routines (Casey et al. 1986), and clinicians would be remiss in neglecting to assess caregiver level of coping with the injury, as well as the potential financial burden (e.g., medical bills and lost time at work) associated with the injury. As an aside, Ganesalingam et al. (2008) found that family burden and distress, though lower in mild TBI, was related to positive LOC at the time of injury. And as illustrated by the parent above who raised concern that her son "hit his brain," it is not at all surprising that concussion can be perceived as a traumatic and stressful event for patients and caregivers alike. Vigilant monitoring of all aspects (direct and indirect) on the part of the clinician is essential in facilitating recovery and minimizing the possibility of persistent symptoms.

8.4 Summary of Research Findings

The DSM-IV and ICD-10 diagnostic criteria are insufficient tools for diagnosing concussion and measuring symptom severity. Fortunately, research is moving toward developing and employing concussion symptom inventories for use in pediatric concussion, and these instruments are continuing to gain popularity as they are refined to improve sensitivity and specificity. Neuropsychological and computer neurocognitive test scores in the absence of additional data can often be misleading, and there continues to be a need for comprehensive evaluation to include the collection of background information, reports from caregivers, teachers and trainers, various rating scales, and appropriate neuropsychological testing. The latter combination is becoming the gold standard in managing the long-term symptoms of concussion.

8.5 Key Points

The vast majority of concussion patients should expect a full recovery within the first 3 months if not sooner of the initial injury. A subset of children will have persistent symptoms and the astute clinician needs to be mindful of the potential for persistent physical, emotional, and/or cognitive complaints.

Controversy exists around the etiology of PCS and PPCS. While there is support for both psychogenic and neurophysiologic contributions, it is incumbent upon all clinicians to conceptualize current complaints in the context of developmental history, premorbid level of cognitive functioning, and prior neuropsychiatric functioning, as children with premorbid issues in these areas are at higher risk for persistent symptoms.

Researchers and clinicians are in general agreement that multiple concussions are associated with increased risk for long-term neurocognitive and emotional/behavioral sequelae.

Ongoing assessment plays an integral role in the development of individually tailored and meaningful treatment plans for patients with persistent symptoms, and these plans need to emphasize return to academic, community, social, and interpersonal endeavors.

Symptom checklists and behavior rating scales have the benefit of reaching teachers and support staff to get a perspective of how the child is managing in their day-to-day environment.

Parent adjustment and response to illness appear directly related to recovery, and routine formal or informal check-in with caregivers is an essential component in the general management of concussion.

References

Achenbach, T. M. (1978). The classification of child psychopathology: A review and analysis of empirical efforts. *Psychological Bulletin, 85*, 1275–1301.

Alexander, M. P. (1995). Mild traumatic brain injury: the Pathophysiology, natural history, and clinical management. *Neurology, 45*, 1253–1260.

Ayr, L. K., Yeates, K. O., Taylor, H. G., & Browne, M. (2009). Dimensions of postconcussive symptoms in children with mild traumatic brain injuries. *Journal of the International Neuropsychological Society, 15*, 19–30.

Bigler, E. D. (2008). Neuropsychology and clinical neuroscience of persistent post-concussive syndrome. *Journal of the International Neuropsychological Society, 14*, 1–22.

Boake, C., McCauley, S. R., Levin, H. S., et al. (2005). Diagnostic criteria for postconcussional syndrome after mild to moderate traumatic brain injury. *The Journal of Neuropsychiatry and Clinical Neurosciences, 17*, 350–356.

Carroll, L. J., Cassidy, J. D., Peloso, P. M., et al. (2004). WHO Collaborating Centre Task Force on Mild Traumatic Brain Injury. *Journal of Rehabilitation Medicine, 43*, 84–105.

Casey, R., Ludwig, S., & McCormick, M. C. (1986). Morbidity following minor head trauma in children. *Pediatrics, 78*, 497–502.

Fann, J., Uomoto, J. M., & Katon, W. J. (2001). Cognitive improvement with treatment of depression following mild traumatic brain injury. *Psychosomatics, 42*, 48–54.

Field, M., Collins, M. W., Lovell, M. R., & Maroon, J. (2003). Does age play a role in recovery from sports-related concussion? A comparison of high school in collegiate athletes. *Journal of Pediatrics, 142*, 546–553.

Ganesalingam, K., Yeates, K. O., Ginn, M. S., et al. (2008). Family burden and parental distress following mild traumatic brain injury in children and its relationship to post-concussive symptoms. *Journal of Pediatric Psychology, 33*(6), 621–629.

Gioia, G. A., Schneider, J. C., Vaughan, C. G., et al. (2009). Which symptom assessments and approaches are uniquely appropriate for paediatric concussion? *British Journal of Sports Medicine, 43*, i13–i22.

Guskiewicz, K. M., Bruce, S. L., Cantu, R. C., Ferrara, M. S., et al. (2004). National Athletic Trainers' Association Position Statement: management of sport-related concussion. *Journal of Athletic Training, 39*, 280–297.

Hall, R. C., Hall, R. C., & Chapman, M. J. (2005). Definition, diagnosis, and forensic implications of postconcussional syndrome. *Psychosomatics, 46*(3), 195–202.

Iverson, G. L. (2005). Outcome from mild traumatic brain injury. *Current Opinions in Psychiatry, 18*, 301–317.

Iverson, G. L., Brooks, B. L., Collins, M. W., & Lovell, M. R. (2006). Tracking neuropsychological recovery following concussion in sport. *Brain Injury, 20*, 245–252.

McCrea, M. A. (2008). *Mild traumtic brain injury and postconcussion syndrome: the new evidence base for diagnosis and treatment.* New York: Oxford Univeristy Press.

McCrory, P. (2001). Does second impact syndrome exists? *Clinical Journal of Sport Medicine, 11*, 144–149.

Miller, L. J., & Mittenberg, W. (1998). Brief cognitive behavioral interventions in mild traumatic brain injury. *Applied Neuropsychology, 5*(4), 172–183.

Mittenberg, W., Wittner, M. S., & Miller, L. J. (1997). Postconcussion syndrome occurs in children. *Neuropsychology, 11*(3), 447–452.

Ommaya, A. K., & Gennarelli, T. A. (1974). Cerebral concussion and traumatic unconsciousness. *Brain, 97*, 633–654.

Ponsford, J. (2005). Rehabilitation interventions after mild head injury. *Current Opinions in Neurology, 18*, 692–697.

Randolph, C., Millis, S., Barr, W. B., McCrea, M., Guskiewicz, K. M., Hammeke, T. A., et al. (2009). Concussion symptom inventory: an empirically derived scale for monitoring resolution of symptoms following sport-related concussion. *Archives of Clinical Neuropsychology, 24*(3), 219–229.

Stovner, L. J., Schrader, H., Mickeviciene, D., Surkiene, D., & Sand, T. (2009). Headache after concussion. *European Journal of Neurology, 16*(1), 112–120.

Yarnell, P. R. (1970). Retrograde memory immediately after concussion. *Lancet, 1*, 863–864.

Yeates, K. O., Luria, J., Bartkowski, H., Rusin, J., Martin, L., & Bigler, E. D. (1999). Postconcussive symptoms in children with mild closed head injuries. *The Journal of Head Trauma Rehabilitation, 14*(4), 337–350.

Yeates, K. O., & Taylor, H. G. (2005). Neurobehavioural outcomes of mild head injury in children and adolescents. *Pediatric Rehabilitation, 8*(1), 5–16.

Chapter 9
Long-Term Treatment of Concussion

Monique S. Burton

9.1 Postconcussion Syndrome

Postconcussion syndrome (PCS) occurs in a small percentage of athletes and other individuals following concussion. About 80% of high school athletes with concussion will recover within 3 weeks (Collins et al. 2006); however, some athletes go on to experience a prolonged recovery.

Several definitions of PCS exist but typically refer to patients with traumatic brain injury (TBI), and scant literature is available regarding PCS in athletes. The World Health Organization (1992) defines PCS as a syndrome that occurs following head trauma (usually sufficiently severe to result in loss of consciousness), and three of the following symptoms must be present: headache, dizziness, fatigue, irritability, difficulty in concentrating or performing mental tasks, impairment of memory, insomnia, and reduced tolerance to stress, emotional excitement or alcohol. With the ICD-10 update, there is no longer indication of how long symptoms must be present to consider a diagnosis of PCS (WHO).

Diagnostic and Statistical Manual of Mental Disorders, Fourth Edition (DSM IV) defines PCS as a history of traumatic brain injury and the presence of at least three of following eight symptoms that persist for at least 3 months: fatigue, sleep disturbance, headache, vertigo/dizziness, irritability, anxiety or depression, personality changes, and apathy. Symptoms must begin or worsen after injury, must interfere with social or occupational functioning, may not be consistent with dementia, and are not better explained by other mental disorders (American Psychiatric Association 2000).

M.S. Burton (✉)
Sports Medicine Program, Seattle Children's Hospital,
Department of Pediatrics and Orthopedics and Sports Medicine,
University of Washington, Seattle, WA, USA
e-mail: monique.burton@seattlechildrens.org

J.N. Apps and K.D. Walter (eds.), *Pediatric and Adolescent Concussion:*
Diagnosis, Management and Outcomes, DOI 10.1007/978-0-387-89545-1_9,
© Springer Science+Business Media, LLC 2012

A definition that may be more relevant to the athletic population is the persistence of cognitive, physical, and/or emotional symptoms of concussion for a time frame longer than normally expected with acknowledgment that symptoms persisting anywhere between 1 and 6 weeks may be adequate for diagnosis of sports-related PCS (Jotwani and Harmon 2010).

9.2   Risk Factors

There is no way to predict which patients that sustain a concussion will go on to have PCS. There are some potential risk factors that may contribute to prolonged PCS, which could help providers recognize those patients that are more likely to experience a protracted recovery. Prolonged PCS have been found to be more likely in athletes with history of previous concussions (Guskiewicz et al. 2003) and concussion occurring at a younger age (Field et al. 2003).

Loss of consciousness, previously used as an indication of severity in grading, occurs in less than 10% of sports related concussions (Guskiewicz et al. 2000), and has not proven to be a predictor of prolonged recovery. A study by Collins et al. reported that in 78 sports related concussions, the presence of amnesia, not loss of consciousness, was predictive of symptoms and neurocognitive deficits following concussion. Athletes that report more symptoms and decreased memory functioning were 10 times more likely to have retrograde amnesia and four times more likely to have anterograde amnesia (Collins et al. 2003b). Asplund et al. found that prolonged recovery or more severe injury may be associated with headache greater than 3 hours, retrograde amnesia, or loss of consciousness (Asplund et al. 2004).

9.3   Treatment Approaches

Concussion symptoms typically improve over time with cognitive and physical rest. Aside from education regarding rest and the recovery process, there are no specific treatment options for concussion (Hunt and Asplund 2010).

Management of prolonged PCS is directed at minimizing the overall symptom profile by treating the predominant complaints. This can be quite challenging since symptoms may both overlap and result in other experienced symptoms, making it difficult to determine the underlying primary cause. For example, difficulty concentrating and focusing may result in headache, irritability, and frustration, or vice versa. It can be helpful for patients to keep a journal of their symptoms with associated details, including when they occur, exacerbating and alleviating factors and progression of other symptoms, to provide guidance for the treatment plan.

Pharmacotherapy has not been found to be particularly successful for prolonged PCS and has primarily been investigated in patients with severe brain injuries (McCrory 2002). However, medications may be helpful in reducing symptoms and improving daily function in patients with PCS. Selection of medications should focus on the management of specific identifiable symptoms and/or modify underlying pathophysiology of the condition with the goal of shortening the duration of symptoms (Hunt and Asplund 2010). Careful consideration needs to be taken when treating athletes with medication for sports concussion, especially in regard to potential side effects and age of patient.

Although considerable overlap exists, post concussion symptoms are often categorized into somatic, emotional, cognitive, and sleep disturbance complaints and are discussed in this format below.

9.3.1 Somatic

Somatic post concussion symptoms include headaches, nausea, vomiting, dizziness, balance problems, fatigue/low energy, visual changes, and photo/phonophobia. Postconcussion headaches are the most common complaint, reported as high as 86% in athletes with sports related head trauma (Guskiewicz et al. 2000). Headaches are often associated with other symptomatology. Collins et al. (2003a) found that high school athletes with postconcussion headaches 7 days postinjury also experienced a larger number of postconcussion symptoms, demonstrated worse performance on reaction time and memory function on neuropsychological testing, and were more likely to have demonstrated on-field anterograde amnesia.

Identification of the type of headache is helpful to guide the most appropriate treatment. The most common types include tension, migraines, cluster, fatigue and mixed posttraumatic headaches. Cervicogenic headaches may be present as well when the mechanism of injury includes a whiplash type of movement (Sabini and Reddy 2010). Migraine variant headaches may occur as an exacerbation of preexisting migraines, first occurrence in predisposed individuals, or of new postconcussion onset.

Over the counter and prescription anti-inflammatories may be helpful, especially with cervicogenic and tension-type headaches. A short course of therapy is recommended to avoid potential rebound effects, particularly when using ibuprofen or other nonsteroidal anti-inflammatories. Amitriptyline is often considered for treatment of postconcussion headaches, especially tension and migraine type; however, effectiveness has been inconsistent. The dose should start low and titrate up as indicated. Beta blockers have been used for headache prophylaxis as well; however, they are not compatible with most athletic participation and need to be discontinued before returning to most sports (Sabini and Reddy 2010). Triptans may be considered for migraine variant headaches.

Dizziness and balance complaints are quite common as well. Although minimal research exists, evaluation by a trained vestibular therapist may be helpful for individuals that express this as their primary and/or persistent complaint. Vestibular therapy may have a greater benefit in the pediatric population than with adults (Alsalaheen et al. 2010).

Table 9.1 Academic accommodations for the concussed student–athlete

- Attendance
  - Excuse absences after the injury
  - Begin at ¼ to ½ days and progress to full days as tolerated
  - If symptoms increase at school, allow to visit/rest in school nurse's office or go home
- Classes
  - Sit in front to minimize distractions
  - Avoid gym class and shop or technical education class
  - Recommend resting, receiving tutoring or an additional study hall instead of "watching" gym class
  - Avoid loud classes, such as music and band
  - Avoid the loud lunchroom, and allow to eat in a quiet area
- Homework
  - Reduce homework load
  - Allow extra time to complete all work
  - Have instructors send written instructions for all assignments home
  - Utilize the teacher's notes or a classmate's notes
  - Allow for tutoring
  - Allow time to catch-up on missed material
- Testing
  - Postpone testing, especially standardized testing
  - Consider open-book or open-note testing
  - Allow extra time to complete tests

Physical therapy should be considered in patients with associated injuries once acute symptoms have declined. Modified progression of rehabilitation exercises may be indicated to prevent exacerbation of symptoms. Addressing injuries will decrease possible misinterpretation and unnecessary treatment of symptoms that may be related to musculoskeletal injury, such as cervicogenic pain causing headache symptoms.

9.3.2 Cognitive Impairment

Cognitive impairment is a common and frustrating post concussion symptoms. Patients complain of "feeling in a fog," difficulty concentrating and remembering, and cognitive fatigue. Cognitive fatigue may be the underlying etiology of postconcussion headaches in some individuals, which when treated appropriately may eliminate headaches symptoms as well (Sabini and Reddy 2010).

The adverse impact of prolonged PCS on school can be quite extensive and challenging. Early notification of an individual's concussion symptoms to teachers, the school counselor and nurse is important, to establish accommodations and reduce chances of falling too far behind in school which may cause increased emotional stress. A letter outlining some general recommendations may be helpful to give some guidance to school personnel (Table 9.1).

If more formal or prolonged accommodations are needed, a Section 504 plan (civil rights entitlement to ensure nondiscrimination of students with disabilities) may be useful. In few cases of significant impairment, an Individualized Education Plan (tailored education plan through the special education system) may be initiated (Kirkwood et al. 2006).

Formal neuropsychological evaluation, preferably by someone with experience with PCS, is an important component in the care of patients with prolonged cognitive symptoms. Although computerized neuropsychological testing is a useful tool in managing patients with sports related concussion, formal neuropsychological evaluation (see Chaps. 8 and 10) is more appropriate for patients with prolonged symptoms. Formal neuropsychological evaluation allows for a detailed assessment of cognitive functioning and additional deficits. The results are helpful for determining appropriate school modifications and guiding cognitive rehabilitation, if indicated. In addition, neuropsychological evaluation may be helpful to distinguish whether or not symptoms, especially of headache, are related to cognitive impairment or chronic headaches. The broad approach in a typical neuropsychological evaluation can also help identify other issues that may be causing symptoms, such as anxiety and depression.

Cognitive rehabilitation has been widely used in severe brain injury, and may be useful in patients with prolonged sports concussion symptoms; however, currently there is not conclusive data to support this (Comper et al. 2005). Treatment focuses on treating specific cognitive deficits. Some evidence exists that neuropsychological test performance improves with neurocognitive rehab; however, it is also felt that changes may be attributed to practice effect (Comper et al. 2005). Although, even this type of improvement in test performance could indicate substantive positive change, in that the patient has the ability to acquire new skills through rehabilitation and exposures to assessment.

Medications are not typically necessary for symptoms of postconcussion cognitive impairment. However, in select patients with prolonged neurocognitive impairment as their primary complaint, neurostimulants may be helpful. Amantadine is a water-soluble salt capable of penetrating the blood–brain barrier, which increases dopamine levels and has been found to be effective in neurobehavioral sequelae in several conditions such as non-Parkinson dementia, Friedreich's ataxia and multiple sclerosis. A small study showed improved cognitive and physical function with amantadine in traumatic brain injury patients (Nickels et al. 1994). Other neurostimulants, such as methylphenidate and atomoxetine, may improve cognitive function and could be considered. Careful consideration should be made in selecting a medication in regard to preexisting conditions as well as potential side effects.

9.3.3 Emotional

Emotional symptoms are not uncommon for athletes and other individuals to experience following concussion. A combination of the concussion itself as well as frustration related to loss of regular sports routine, identity as an athlete, and social interactions related to sports may lead to depression and/or anxiety, especially when recovery is prolonged or discontinuation of sport is advised. Patients may report irritability, sadness, emotional liability, and/or anxiety. Observation for these symptoms as well as changes in usual behavior, atypical responses to regular events, and personality changes should be monitored for by family members/caregivers and friends as well as the health care provider.

Management approaches should include a thorough mental health history, including premorbid psychiatric conditions and family history, as well as evaluation for concomitant symptoms such as cognitive fatigue and overstimulation, which may overlap with depressive symptoms but resolve when addressed appropriately. If injured patients have preexisting mental health disorders or risk factors for mental health disorders, a recommendation to initiate psychotherapy or increase psychotherapy visits while symptomatic would be encouraged. For those whom initial treatment recommendations include counseling, they should be encouraged to work with a sports psychologist or Cognitive-Behavioral psychologist familiar with concussions. Cognitive-Behavioral Therapy is a manualized treatment approach shown to be effective in the treatment of various emotional issues, including anxiety and depression, with some support for utilizing the approach in brain injuries, including concussion (Mittenberg et al. 1996).

In selective cases, especially when emotional symptoms are prolonged, medications may be useful. Selective serotonin reuptake inhibitors (SSRI), including sertraline, citalopram, and fluoxetine, are often considered for patients with symptoms of depression and/or anxiety. Treatment with SSRIs may help decrease psychological distress, including anger, aggression, and difficulty with normal functioning as well as other post concussion symptoms, such as headache, dizziness, and blurred vision (Fann et al. 2000). Mood stabilizers could be considered for patients with emotional lability.

9.3.4   Sleep Disturbance

Sleep disturbances, including either hypersomnolence or insomnia, are common following injury. Sleep hygiene education is the first line of therapy and should be discussed early in concussion management to help reduce associated symptoms. Recommendations include attempting a normal sleep schedule of going to bed and waking up at regular times and eliminating distractions such as computers, TV, video games, and cell phones from the bedroom. In addition, napping should be minimized to no more than 30 min, and caffeine consumption should be avoided in late afternoon or evening. Alcohol, drug use, and nicotine should also be avoided. In refractory cases, medications may be considered, including melatonin, trazodone, amitriptyline, nortriptyline, and ramelteon (Sabini and Reddy 2010). Undesired side effects and cognitive impairment may result from benzodiazepines, antihistamine, and anticholinergic medications and therefore should be avoided.

9.4   Other Considerations

Recognizing that prolonged injury recovery can have a significant impact on a child or teen's social functioning is an important component of this complex treatment planning. Often recommendations may need to include suggestions for additional extracurricular activities in which the individual can participate but that will not exacerbate symptoms or place them at unnecessary risk for additional injury. This can include remaining involved with sports clubs in a different, nonathletic capacity such as being a student manager, joining new clubs or organizations, or engaging in other tasks in which they might excel.

Adjunctive therapies have not been well studied, but may be useful in the management of PCS. Massage therapy, including craniosacral therapy, may be helpful in patients with muscular dysfunction from associated injuries related to the mechanism of the concussion. In addition, it may provide relaxation from both physical and emotional stress associated with prolonged symptoms which may assist with alleviating other symptoms. Acupuncture and chiropractic care have not been well studied in relation to sports concussion, but may be useful in treating related symptoms and should be considered.

9.4.1   Subsymptom Threshold Exercise

Preliminary studies suggest subsymptom threshold exercise may be beneficial in the treatment of prolonged PCS. Leddy et al. demonstrated symptom level and length of exercise ability improved with a controlled program of subsymptom threshold exercise (Leddy et al. 2010). In another study involving children, a gradual, closely supervised active rehabilitation program after the acute period of one month resulted in significant and rapid improvement of symptoms and an ability to return to normal lifestyles and sport participation (Gagnon et al. 2009).

9.5   Conclusions

Prolonged symptoms following concussion represent a very frustrating and challenging experience. Specific treatment options currently are limited and effectiveness varies. Establishment of a supportive environment is very important to help young athletes and individuals cope with this situation. While limited data exist to help make long-term treatment decisions for children and adolescents with PCS, neuropsychological evaluation can be helpful in establishing a treatment plan. Treating symptoms may include medications for appropriate somatic complaints, therapy such as Cognitive-Behavioral Therapy for emotional concerns, continuous patient and family education and support, and consideration of adjunctive therapies.

Providing recommendations for alternative activities during this time period can be helpful, including involvement, with their sports team as a manager or student coach, or trying other new extracurricular activities that do not exacerbate symptoms. Regular sports psychology visits to address frustrations and questions regarding their concussion may be helpful as well.

9.6 Key Points

The majority of patients recover from concussion symptoms within 3 weeks.

Risk factors for prolonged concussion symptoms include number of previous concussions, younger age, and amnesia.

Postconcussion headaches are the most common long-term complaint.

No specific treatment exists for prolonged post concussion symptoms, so management of PCS should focus on targeting specific identifiable symptoms.

Education regarding recovery process is an important part of management.

Formal neuropsychological testing may be a useful tool in concussion management.

Medication therapy should be reserved for symptoms that are prolonged and create significant impairment, usually after nonmedical therapies have failed.

Adjunctive therapies might be considered as part of the treatment plan, including physical therapy, massage, acupuncture, and chiropractic care.

References

American Psychiatric Association. (2000). Diagnostic and statistical manual of mental disorders (4th ed.). Text Revision. DSM-IV-TR. Washington, DC: APA.

Alsalaheen, B. A., Mucha, A., Morris, L. O., Whitney, S. L., Furman, J. M., & Camiolo-Reddy, C. E. (2010). Vestibular rehabilitation for dizziness and balance disorders after concussion. *J Neurol Phys Ther, 34*(2), 87–93.

Asplund, C. A., McKeag, D. B., & Olsen, C. H. (2004). Sports-related concussion: factors associated with prolonged return to play. *Clinical Journal of Sport Medicine, 14*, 339–343.

Collins, M. W., Field, M., Lovell, M. R., Iverson, G., Johnston, K. M., & Maroon, J. (2003a). Relationship between postconcussion headache and neuropsychological test performance in high school athletes. *The American Journal of Sports Medicine, 31*(2), 168–173.

Collins, M. W., Iverson, G. L., Lovell, M. R., McKeag, D. B., Norwig, J., & Maroon, J. (2003b). On-field predictors of neuropsychological and symptom deficit following sports-related concussion. *Clinical Journal of Sport Medicine, 13*, 222–229.

Collins, M., Lovell, M., Iverson, G. Ide, T., & Maroon, J. (2006). Examining concussion rates and return to play in high school football players wearing newer helmet technology: a three-year prospective cohort study. *Neurosurgery, 58*(2), 275–286.

Comper, P., Bisschop, S. M., Cardine, N., & Tricco, A. (2005). A systematic review of treatments for mild traumatic brain injury. *Brain Injury, 19*(11), 863–880.

Fann, J. R., Uomoto, J. M., & Katon, W. J. (2000). Sertraline in treatment of major depression following mild traumatic brain injury. *The Journal of Neuropsychiatry and Clinical Neurosciences, 12*(2), 226–232.

Field, M., Collins, M. W., Lovell, M. R., & Maroon, J. (2003). Does age play a role in recovery from sports-related concussion? A comparison of high school and collegiate athletes. *Journal of Pediatrics, 142*, 446–553.

Gagnon, I., Galli, C., Friedman, D., Grilli, L., & Iverson, G. L. (2009). Active rehabilitation for children who are slow to recover following sport-related concussion. *Brain Injury, 23*(12), 956–964.

Guskiewicz, K. M., McCrea, M., Marshall, S. W., Cantu, R. C., Randolph, C., & Barr, W. (2003). Cumulative effects associated with recurrent concussion in collegiate football players: the NCAA concussion study. *Journal of American Medical Association, 290*(19), 2549–2555.

Guskiewicz K. Weaver, N. L., Padua, D. A., & Garrett, W. E. (2000). Epidemiology of concussion in collegiate and high school football players. *The American Journal of Sports Medicine, 28*, 643–650.

Hunt, T., & Asplund, C. (2010). Concussion assessment and management. *Clinics in Sports Medicine, 29*, 5–17.

Jotwani, V., & Harmon, K. G. (2010). Postconcussion syndrome in athletes. *Current Sports Medicine Reports, 9*(1), 21–26.

Kirkwood, M. W., Yeates, K. O., & Wilson, P. E. (2006). Pediatric sport-related concussion: a review of the clinical management of an oft-neglected population. *Pediatrics, 117*(4), 1359–1371.

Leddy, J. L., Kozlowski, K., Donnelly, J. P., Pendergast, D. R., Epstein, L. H., & Willer, B. (2010). A preliminary study of subsymptom threshold exercise training for refractory post-concussion syndrome. *Clinical Journal of Sport Medicine, 20*(1), 21–27.

McCrory, P. (2002). Should we treat concussion pharmacologically? The need for evidence based pharmacological treatment for the concussed athlete. *British Journal of Sports Medicine, 36*(1), 3–5.

Mittenberg, W., Tremont, G., Zielinski, R. E., Fichera, S., & Rayls, K. R. (1996). Cognitive-Behavioral prevention of postconsussion syndrome. *Archives of Clinical Neuropsychology, 11*(2), 139–145.

Nickels, J. L., Schneider, W. N., Dombovy, M. L., & Wong, T. M. (1994). Clinical use of amantadine in brain injury rehabilitation. *Brain Injury, 8*(8), 709–718.

Sabini, R. C., & Reddy, C. C. (2010). Concussion management and treatment considerations in the adolescent population. *The Physician and SportsMedicine, 38*(1), 139–146.

World Health Organization. (1992). *The ICD-10 Classification of Mental and Behavioural Disorders: Clinical Descriptions and Diagnostic Guidelines*. Geneva, Switzerland: WHO.

Chapter 10
Methods of Formal Neurocognitive Assessment of Concussion

Nathan E. Kegel and Mark R. Lovell

10.1 Introduction

Traumatic brain injury (TBI) is the leading cause of acquired disability in children in the United States. Much like statistics cited elsewhere in this text, the Centers for Disease Control and Prevention estimates nearly 475,000 children between the age of 0 and 14 are treated for TBI in emergency departments annually (CDC 2010), with as many as 90% of TBI being classified as "mild" (McCrea 2008). Pediatric mild traumatic brain injury (mTBI), or concussion, is frequently associated with neuropsychological impairments that can adversely affect cognitive, academic, behavioral, and interpersonal functioning. This chapter reviews methods of formal assessment of pediatric concussion, with an emphasis on neuropsychological and neurocognitive assessment. Critical research related to neurocognitive assessment of pediatric concussion is reviewed and implications of research findings are discussed. Recent advances in the assessment of pediatric concussion are presented.

10.1.1 Definition of Concussion

The definition of concussion has changed considerably over the past several decades as a result of increasing awareness and understanding gained through research and practice. Similar to definitions quoted elsewhere in this text, concussion, as currently presented in the 2008 "Consensus Statement on Concussion in Sport"

N.E. Kegel (✉) • M.R. Lovell
University of Pittsburgh Medical Center,
Sports Medicine Concussion Program, Pittsburgh, PA, USA
e-mail: kegelne@upmc.edu

J.N. Apps and K.D. Walter (eds.), *Pediatric and Adolescent Concussion:*
Diagnosis, Management and Outcomes, DOI 10.1007/978-0-387-89545-1_10,
© Springer Science+Business Media, LLC 2012

(McCrory et al. 2009) as well as the "CDC Toolkit for Mild TBI" (CDC 2007), is defined as a complex pathophysiological process affecting the brain, induced by traumatic biomechanical forces. It typically involves a rapid onset of symptoms and functional impairments in neurocognitive functioning that resolve spontaneously. Loss of consciousness does not necessarily occur and, in fact, is only present in roughly 10% of concussions (Collins et al. 2003). In addition, standard structural neuroimaging techniques generally do not detect abnormalities (McCrory et al. 2009). The "Consensus Statement on Concussion in Sport" also recognizes the importance of neurocognitive testing in the evaluation and management of concussion.

10.1.2 Background on Neuropsychological Assessment

Neuropsychological research on concussion has helped to identify a constellation of specific neurocognitive difficulties including deficits in sustained attention, executive functioning, reduced processing speed and reaction time, and problems with learning and memory of new information (Iverson et al. 2006). Neurocognitive assessment targeting these areas is an essential component in the postacute stage of pediatric concussion evaluation (Kirkwood et al. 2008). It provides an objective means of assessment that augments the clinical interview, which often relies on subjective reporting of symptoms, and adds increased specificity and prognostic utility to the evaluation and management of concussion (Iverson 2007; Lau et al. 2009; Van Kampen et al. 2006).

The two primary approaches to neuropsychological assessment of concussion are paper and pencil measures and computerized assessment. Traditional paper and pencil tests generally carry well-established reliability and validity and have been shown to be sensitive to the effects of concussion (Collins et al. 1999). However, these types of tests do not lend themselves well to the type of short-term serial assessment often needed when evaluating and managing recovery from concussion, as they often lack alternative forms and are thus susceptible to practice effects. In addition, traditional neuropsychological tests are less able to detect subtle changes in reaction time and processing speed, generally relying on manually operated stopwatches. Computerized neuropsychological test batteries have been developed to address these shortcomings. Several computerized neurocognitive measures have been developed to assess concussion including ImPACT, HeadMinder, and CogSport/AxonSports. ImPACT, and Pediatric ImPACT in particular, is discussed in greater depth later in this chapter, while other computerized assessments are covered elsewhere in the text. These programs offer several advantages to traditional testing including relatively brief administration times (20–30 min), alternative forms to allow for serial tracking of recovery, and computerized timing mechanisms capable of measuring reaction times to the hundredth of a second. Perhaps most importantly, they provide the opportunity for efficient preinjury baseline testing of groups of children. This is particularly relevant to children at higher risk for concussion, such as athletes. Baseline assessments allow clinicians to accurately evaluate the effects of concussion on a child's neurocognitive functioning, and ultimately help to better inform postinjury management.

10.2   Review of Current Research

Research on neuropsychological functioning in pediatric concussion has expanded rapidly over the past decade. A broad range of neurocognitive skills (e.g., memory, attention, inhibition, executive functioning) have been empirically examined using varying methodology to add valuable findings to our understanding of pediatric concussion. Furthermore, functional academic skills and neurobehavioral and social functioning are an important element in pediatric neuropsychological assessment, and these topics have been addressed in the literature. This section presents a broad review of current literature related to neuropsychological assessment of pediatric concussion.

10.2.1   General Intellectual Ability

Traditional IQ tests provide neuropsychologists with information about a wide range of cognitive skills, as well as general estimate of overall cognitive functioning (i.e., full scale IQ). Given their often lengthy administration time and lack of utility as a serial assessment tool, traditional IQ tests are generally not a practical component of postinjury neurocognitive assessment. However, they have been used extensively in research to demonstrate characteristics of overall cognitive functioning following pediatric concussion.

The majority of research on general intellectual ability following concussion has utilized Wechsler scales and focused on long-term outcomes and predictors of neurocognitive functioning. For example, Catroppa and Anderson (2003) examined intellectual skills in mild, moderate, and severe TBI groups 24 months postinjury. The severe TBI group demonstrated the greatest improvement in overall cognitive functioning over 24 months as measured by the Full Scale IQ (FSIQ) index of the *Wechsler Intelligence Scale for Children, Third Edition* (WISC-III). This finding speaks to the fact that the severe TBI group was significantly more impaired in the acute period following the injury (0–3 months). Similar findings were also evident in a longitudinal study with performance on the WISC-III at 6 months, 12 months, and 3–5 years postinjury (Fay et al. 2009). Catroppa and Anderson (2003) also concluded that socioeconomic status (SES) and injury severity were the best predictors of postinjury intellectual functioning, with lower SES and more severe injury associated with poorer intellectual functioning 24 months postinjury.

Long-term consequences of pediatric concussion on general cognitive ability have been examined using both retrospective and longitudinal designs. Horneman and Emanuelson (2009) retrospectively examined cognitive functioning of individuals who had sustained TBI approximately 10 years earlier during childhood. Compared to a healthy control group, the TBI group demonstrated significantly poorer performance on tasks of verbal IQ (e.g., Vocabulary) compared to performance on visual-spatial tasks such as Block Design. This finding was somewhat interesting to the authors and led them to recommend the importance of rehabilitation focusing verbal skills following pediatric head injury.

In a 23-year follow-up study of pediatric head injury, Hessen et al. (2007) examined neurocognitive functioning as it relates to various injury characteristics such as posttraumatic amnesia, EEG findings, and skull fracture. The primary findings indicated that the most important predictor of poor outcome on a measure of cognitive functioning (Norwegian version of the *Wechsler Adult Intelligence Scale*) was length of posttraumatic amnesia. Other studies have also highlighted the importance of both anterograde and posttraumatic amnesia to postinjury neurocognitive functioning and symptom resolution (Cantu 2001; Lovell et al. 2003). Another way to assess the effects of concussion on cognitive functioning at different points in childhood is through the use of a cross-sectional design. Anderson et al. (2000) divided a group of children who sustained TBI into a "young" (i.e., 3–7 years old at injury) and "old" group (i.e., 8–12 years old at injury) and assessed cognitive functioning using the WISC-III. Several interesting findings were revealed based on age group and severity of injury. Moderately and mildly injured children showed a similar increase in cognitive abilities in serial testing, regardless of age group. Among severely injured participants, children in the "old" group demonstrated increased performance with steep curves over the first 12 months postinjury, but the "young" group demonstrated flatter recovery curve, indicating minimal improvement over time.

10.2.2 *Learning and Memory*

Assessment of memory is of particular interest to the postinjury evaluation of pediatric concussion. The most common types of memory tasks utilized fall into two broad categories: general memory via learning tasks and working memory. List learning tasks, such as the *California Verbal Learning Test-Children's Version* (CVLT-C) are frequently used to assess verbal learning and memory. Working memory involves holding information in an active state to utilize it for future goal-oriented action. It can be examined using reverse digit span tests and letter-number sequencing tasks where random letters and numbers must be held in memory then mentally manipulated according to rules of the task. Research related to memory functioning has provided information regarding short-term deficits and long-term prognosis following pediatric concussion.

List learning tasks are useful in identifying several aspects of memory including initial acquisition, consolidation, and retrieval following a delay. Comparison of children with TBI with healthy controls has indicated difficulty with initial encoding on verbal learning tasks for the TBI group (Mandalis et al. 2007). This study did not find differences between TBI and control groups in consolidation or retrieval learning patterns. The difficulties with initial encoding found by Mandalis et al. (2007) are particularly relevant to children's academic performance, and may indicate the need for increased repetition of information in the classroom.

Conklin et al. (2008) assessed working memory in a group of children using a performance-based task, reverse digit span, and an ecologically valid parent rating scale, the *Behavior Rating Inventory of Executive Function* (BRIEF). Comparisons of children with TBI and healthy controls indicated impairments on both measures. However, there was no statistical association between performance- and parent-based measures of working memory. Other studies have also failed to establish relationships between performance-based measures and rating scales (Anderson et al. 2002; Vriezen and Pigott 2002). It is likely that the reverse digit span task and the Working Memory index of the BRIEF examine slightly different aspects of working memory, with both forms of assessment providing equally valuable information. Ecologically valid measures, such as parent rating scales, should not be neglected in the pediatric concussion evaluation as they can provide useful information about the child's functioning in the natural environment.

In a longitudinal follow-up study 5 years postchildhood TBI, Anderson and Catroppa (2007) employed a number of memory tasks to determine the effects of TBI. Expected differences between the TBI group and control group were not found on a measure of simple visual memory (e.g., block span task) or working memory (e.g., reverse digit span task). When examining the severity of TBI, several interesting results emerged. Children with severe TBI performed more poorly than controls on both spontaneous and delayed recall for a list-learning task. Additionally, the mild TBI group outperformed the severe TBI group on delayed recall. The expected relationship between TBI severity and decreased visual-spatial memory performance was not supported. Overall, it appeared that simple, automatic immediate memory processes may be largely unaffected by childhood TBI, while deficits in complex auditory-verbal memory were apparent as injury severity increased.

10.2.3   Attention

Deficits in attentional capacity following concussion can have a negative impact on a child's academic, adaptive, and social functioning. Attention is a complex construct that is often broken down into component processes, such as sustained and shifting attention, during assessment. Park et al. (2009) took a component process approach when examining factors of attention and their ability to predict severity of brain injury. For example, sustained attention was assessed via the *Conners' Continuous Performance Test – II* (CPT-II), while shifting attention was examined using the Digit Symbol Coding and Symbol Search subtests of the WISC-III. Children with TBI performed significantly worse than healthy controls on all measures of attention. Only shifting attention, as measured by the Coding and Symbol Search subtests of the WISC-III, and focused attention, as measured by Trail Making Tests Part A and B, were significant predictors of TBI severity.

Catroppa and Anderson (2005) examined sustained, selective, and shifting attention at several points over a 2-year period following TBI. Several interesting findings emerged when comparing the different components of attention and severity of injury. Children with severe TBI achieved fewer correct responses on measures of sustained attention, had problems working efficiently over time, and showed a gradual increase in errors. Over time, the severe TBI group generally responded more quickly and impulsively. On tasks measuring selective and shifting attention, the severe TBI group exhibited the most significant initial impairment, but also demonstrated the steepest recovery curve. Overall, deficits in attention for the TBI group appeared to persist to the 2-year follow-up on tasks relying on speed and visuomotor coordination.

In order to examine the impact of age at the time of injury, Fenwick and Anderson (1999) assessed a group of children using standardized measures of sustained, focused, and divided attention. Results indicated that early-injured children performed significantly worse than later-injury children. In other words, children who were older at the point at which they sustained their TBI were more likely to demonstrate intact attentional skills. However, overall, both younger and older children in the TBI group performed more poorly than controls. These results are particularly important when considering long-term prognosis. A child who sustains a head injury at a young age may be more prone to deficits in attention that may negatively affect academic and social functioning.

Children with concussion often exhibit acquired attention problems that present in a similar manner to a clinical diagnosis of Attention-Deficit/Hyperactivity Disorder (ADHD) (Yeates et al. 2005). Additionally, Yeates et al. (2005) found that children with a premorbid history of ADHD often exhibit more pronounced long-term behavioral, but not cognitive, difficulties. These findings highlight the importance of gathering a detailed premorbid history during the clinical interview. Knowing a child has a premorbid history of attention problems or ADHD can be an important factor in determining prognosis and recovery time in pediatric concussion.

10.2.4 Executive Functioning

Executive functioning is a cognitive construct used to describe an individual's ability to maintain an appropriate problem solving set to guide future (goal-directed) behavior (Tsatsanis 2005). Executive functioning consists of specific skills including cognitive flexibility, inhibition, planning, organization, and self-monitoring, some of which are related or dependent upon one another. These higher order processes are generally presumed to be mediated by the prefrontal cortex, and are particularly vulnerable following TBI. Given the long-term developmental course of executive functioning, generally thought to continue into early adulthood, the consequences of TBI may not be realized for years after the injury. The complexity and developmental course of executive functioning, not to mention its importance to academic and adaptive functioning, make it an interesting construct to address in pediatric concussion research.

Slomine et al. (2002) used a prospective design to examine associations between components of executive functioning and age at injury, injury severity, and neuro-anatomical variables for children who sustained TBI. Younger age at injury was found to be associated with poorer performance on tests assessing the ability to categorize, shift cognitive strategy, and generate new information. Frontal lesion volume was not associated with any of the executive function measures. However, extrafrontal lesion and a higher total number of lesions were associated with the ability to generate novel information. These neuroanatomical findings may relate to the fact that many frontal executive processes are mediated by other parts of the brain, and disruptions of connections to other critical areas may negatively impact test performance.

Various components of executive functioning have been examined longitudinally using a number of different measures. Anderson and Catroppa (2005) found significant effects for severity of TBI on planning, goal setting, and problem-solving at a 2-year follow-up. On a simple task of cognitive flexibility, the TBI group was able to perform comparably in terms of accuracy, but took significantly longer to complete the task. Other long-term longitudinal studies, ranging from 5 to 10 years, have suggested mixed evidence based on injury severity over time (Muscara et al. 2008; Nadebaum et al. 2007). In general, severely injured children tend to show impaired performance on measures of cognitive flexibility and goal setting. Additionally, behavioral ratings of executive function tend to be more impaired for children with severe TBI (Nadebaum et al. 2007).

Response inhibition is another component of executive functioning that is often assessed via classic go/no-go tasks where the examinee must quickly provide a simple response based on stimuli. Inhibition has been shown to be impaired immediately following TBI, with an improvement by 2 years postinjury (Leblanc et al. 2005). In addition, Leblanc et al. (2005) found that younger TBI patients were initially more impaired, but exhibited a greater recovery than older TBI patients.

Given the lack of ecological validity of some lab-based measures of executive functioning, Chevignard et al. (2009) attempted to measure using a naturalistic task in conjunction with a behavioral rating scale completed by the parent. On the naturalistic task of executive function, which incorporated elements of planning and multitasking, all quantitative and qualitative variables were significantly impaired for the TBI group. In addition, Chevignard and colleagues found that both the naturalistic task and parent ratings of executive functioning were shown to be more sensitive to executive functioning deficits. Executive functioning is often difficult to cleanly assess, and sometimes does not correlate with real world outcomes. Thus, naturalistic assessment, and certainly behavioral ratings, can be important sources of information when evaluating pediatric concussion.

10.2.5 Functional Outcomes

Thus far we have outlined research revealing notable deficits in neurocognitive functioning following pediatric concussion. Traditional neuropsychological assessment has highlighted difficulties in various neurocognitive skills such as attention, memory, and executive functioning. The impact of these postinjury deficits inevitably manifest in the child's natural environment. Pediatric concussion can result in widespread academic difficulties, maladaptive behavior problems, and disrupted social functioning. A thorough neuropsychological evaluation can address these concerns during parent and child interview, through school consultation, or by having parents and teachers complete rating scales. This section reviews recent research examining functional outcomes following pediatric concussion.

10.2.5.1 Academic

Concussion can potentially have an impact on a multitude of academic skills including reading fluency and comprehension, mathematics problem-solving, and organization during writing tasks. Which skills are ultimately affected depends on combinations of variables related to the injury and the child sustaining the injury. Research to date has sought to explore various factors of concussion, or moderate or severe TBI, and their relationship to academic outcomes. Young children who sustained TBI have been shown to carry increased risks for deficits in school readiness skills as measured by reading, writing, and math subtests of the *Woodcock-Johnson Tests of Achievement, 3rd Edition* (WJ-III) (Taylor et al. 2008). In this study, injury severity was related to performance on academic assessments, with more severely injured children performing worse than moderately or mildly injured children.

Miller and Donders (2003) attempted to draw meaningful comparisons between performance on the CVLT-C, a verbal list learning task, and placement in special education classes 2 years postinjury. Results indicated that children who obtained a composite *T*-score of less than 45 on the CVLT-C were 8–13 times more likely to be placed in special education 12–24 months later. In this case, neuropsychological test scores were sensitive to differences in injury severity and also explained a significant portion of the variance in educational outcome following pediatric concussion.

Levin et al. (2001) investigated the effects of head injury on development of word fluency in children. Younger children with severe TBI exhibited less improvement over time than older severely injured children. The authors explained these findings by hypothesizing that TBI at a young age shortens the period of normal brain function during which children can consolidate language functioning, with an end result of decreased performance on word generation tasks under timed conditions.

The ultimate goal of neuropsychological assessment is to inform treatment recommendations. Once acute symptoms of concussion have resolved it is often advisable to begin some form of cognitive rehabilitation. With regard to academic skills, fluency training may be an effective intervention to improve academic performance following pediatric concussion. Chapman et al. (2005) utilized a single subject, multiple baseline design to examine the effects of fluency training on several students with concussion. Fluency training involves over-learning specific skills with the intention of increasing speed and accuracy. All five participants in the study showed significant improvements in simple math calculations and correctly responding to questions. Fluency training may be an effective intervention for teachers working with children recovering from concussion; however, more research is needed in this area.

10.2.5.2   Behavioral

Persistent patterns of maladaptive behavior can be observed several months or even years after TBI (Anderson et al. 2004; Fay et al. 2009). Several studies have attempted to examine risk factors and characteristics of behavioral change following pediatric concussion or more significant TBI. Chapman et al. (2010) assessed children aged 3–7 at 6 months, 12 months, and 18 months postinjury using the *Child Behavior Checklist* (CBCL), a broad behavior rating scale, and the BRIEF. Children who sustained severe TBI exhibited significantly higher rates of new externalizing behavior problems than children with moderate TBI and orthopedic impairment. Permissive parenting, family dysfunction, and SES were notable predictors of the emergence of behavior problems.

Cole et al. (2008) looked specifically at aggressive behavior following severe pediatric TBI using the CBCL and *Overt Aggression Scale* (OAS). Several preinjury risk factors were identified including preexisting aggression, attention problems, and anxiety. Overall, results indicated a significant increase in caregiver ratings of aggressive behavior after TBI. Maladaptive behavior, such as aggression, can be a prominent symptom following TBI, and often interferes with successful treatment. By increasing awareness of risk factors of postinjury aggression, potentially susceptible children can be accurately identified and rehabilitation programs tailored to meet their needs.

10.2.5.3   Social

Much like the development of cognitive and academic skills, social skills development is a critical process that takes place throughout childhood and adolescence. The developmental significance of social skills makes them especially vulnerable to the negative effects of pediatric concussion. Yeates et al. (2004) assessed social skills of children with TBI at several points during the first year postinjury as well as at an extended follow-up 4 years later. The CBCL and *Vineland Adaptive Behavior Scales* (VABS) were used to obtain parent ratings of social skills, while the *Interpersonal Negotiation Strategies* (INS) interview was used as a functional measure of social problem-solving. Overall, children who sustained TBI between 6 and 12 years of age demonstrated poorer social outcomes than children with orthopedic impairment. In addition, findings did not indicate substantial improvement in social functioning over time, and in some cases reflect worsening outcomes.

Several risk factors have been shown to significantly increase negative social outcomes following childhood TBI, most notably age at injury and clinical ratings of injury severity (Wells et al. 2009). A retrospective review of children who sustained TBI in preschool indicated that those less than 4 years old at the time of injury exhibited poorer social outcomes when compared to older preschoolers (Sonnenberg et al. 2010). Assessment of a child's social functioning, preferably from multiple sources, is an important aspect of formal assessment of concussion, and can provide useful directions when designing a postinjury treatment plan.

10.2.6 Summary of Research

The research reviewed in this section highlights recent findings related to neuropsychological assessment of TBI and pediatric concussion. Deficits in neurocognitive functioning are apparent across domains of memory, attention, and executive functioning. In general, more severe injuries tend to lead to more significant neurocognitive deficits. Longitudinal studies revealed improvements over time regardless of injury severity.

Functional outcomes are also an important aspect of a neuropsychological evaluation following pediatric concussion. Children may exhibit a number of functional difficulties following concussion, including problems with academic fluency, aggressive or irritable behavior, and disruption in social functioning. Assessing a child's academic, behavioral, and social functioning provides information that is useful when recommending treatment and designing rehabilitation programs.

10.3 A Model of Pediatric Concussion Assessment

As outlined thus far in this chapter, pediatric concussion can have a negative impact on a child's neurocognitive and neurobehavioral functioning. As such, an ideal model of pediatric concussion assessment should encompass these areas. Gioia et al. (2009) describe a model that includes standardized performance on a measure of neurocognitive functioning as well as structured ratings of symptoms and functional manifestations. In the case of this model, primary measures include *Pediatric Immediate Post-Concussion Assessment and Cognitive Testing* (ImPACT; Lovell et al. 2002), the *Acute Concussion Evaluation* (ACE; Gioia et al. 2008a), and *Post-Concussion Symptom Inventories* (PCSIs). The authors also suggest the additional consideration of the *Multidimensional Fatigue Scale of the Pediatric Quality of Life Scale, Version 4.0* (Varni et al. 2004) to more thoroughly assess fatigue and sleep problem often associated with concussion.

10.3.1   Pediatric ImPACT

The traditional ImPACT neuropsychological test battery (age 11–60) is comprised of six subtests that assess multiple neurocognitive abilities. Cognitive skills that are measured by these subtests range from verbal and visual memory and learning to reaction time. Several subtests incorporate multiple cognitive domains. For example, the X's and O's subtest requires the examinee to hold in memory a visual pattern while completing a choice reaction time test. The reaction time test provides interference within a working memory paradigm. To aid in test interpretation, the clinical report provides composite scores for verbal memory, visual memory, visual motor speed, and reaction time. The test has five alternative versions: a baseline version for preinjury testing and four alternative postinjury versions.

Pediatric ImPACT is an adaptation of the ImPACT battery for children with brain injury aged 5–12 years. It consists of seven subtests that mirror the adolescent/adult version of ImPACT, but present material in a manner that makes it more appealing and valid for children. Content of the subtests includes a story theme to engage children in the task while measuring cognitive abilities. The subtest's content taps several key neurocognitive domains related to concussion including episodic memory for verbal and visual information, working memory, information processing speed, and reaction time. Initial psychometric analyses of the instrument indicate strong developmental age effects, small performance differences between boys and girls, evidence of reasonable subtest internal consistency and test–retest reliability, equivalence among the forms, and performance differences between children with concussion and matched controls (Gioia et al. 2009).

10.3.2   Acute Concussion Evaluation

The ACE (Gioia et al. 2008a) is a systematic evidence-based protocol used to assess mTBI and provide initial follow-up treatment recommendations for patients and their families. The ACE is administered as a clinical interview of the patient directly or knowledgeable caregiver as part of a clinical examination. It is organized into the following areas of inquiry: (1) specific characteristics of the injury including details of the blow to the head, loss of consciousness, or amnesia, (2) a broad range of 22 symptoms and five signs associated with mTBI, referred to as the ACE symptom checklist, and (3) risk factors that may predict prolonged recovery including history of concussion, headaches, learning disability, attention deficit, and anxiety/depression. The ACE has demonstrated adequate to good psychometrics including reliable internal consistency and predictive validity (Gioia et al. 2008a).

10.3.3 *Postconcussion Symptom Inventory*

Symptom inventories allow for a structured assessment of symptoms that augments information gained through neurocognitive assessment. It is preferable to obtain perspectives of multiple respondents including parents, teachers, and the injured child. The pediatric PCSI is an adaptation of the adolescent/adult self-report scale (Gioia et al. 2008b; Lovell et al. 2006). It features a 26-item inventory of observable signs that respondents rate on a 7-point Likert scale. The instructions ask the parent/teacher to rate the extent to which each symptom is observed in the home/school setting. The inventory focuses on the physical, cognitive, and behavioral symptoms commonly seen after concussion. Two forms are administered during the first visit. The first form is a retrospective preinjury baseline report in which the respondent is asked to rate the extent to which any symptoms were present during the days leading up to the injury. The second form focuses on postinjury report of symptoms over the past day since the injury. The postinjury form is then administered at each follow-up visit to track symptom progression. Self-report PCSI forms for children are age-dependent (age 5–7, 8–12, and 13–18 years) and feature content at appropriate reading and vocabulary levels for the various age groups. Current research on these rating scales indicates that parents are reliable reporters of symptoms of their children's concussion and add relevant information above and beyond their children's own symptom reports (Gioia et al. 2008a, b).

10.4 Key Points

Concussion is a pathophysiological process that can result in compromised neurocognitive and neurobehavioral functioning.

Neuropsychological assessment of pediatric concussion provides useful information pertaining to the child's neurocognitive and neurobehavioral functioning.

Evidence from available literature suggests prominent difficulties in memory, attention, and executive functioning following TBI and pediatric concussion.

More severe injuries (i.e., longer intensity and duration of postinjury symptoms) generally result in more impaired neurocognitive and neurobehavioral functioning.

The majority of cases return to normal neurocognitive functioning following recovery from concussion.

An effective model of pediatric concussion assessment incorporates formal neurocognitive assessment with multirespondent symptom/behavioral ratings.

Information gained through the neuropsychological assessment can be used when planning academic, behavioral, and social interventions.

References

Anderson, V., Anderson, P., Northam, E., et al. (2002). Relationships between cognitive and behavioral measures of executive function in children with brain disease. *Child Neuropsychology, 8*, 2231–240.

Anderson, V., & Catroppa, C. (2005). Recovery of executive skills following paediatric traumatic brain injury (TBI): a 2 year follow-up. *Brain Injury, 19*, 459–470.

Anderson, V., & Catroppa, C. (2007). Memory outcome at 5 years post-childhood traumatic brain injury. *Brain Injury, 21*, 1399–1409.

Anderson, V., Catroppa, C., Rosenfeld, J., et al. (2000). Recovery of memory function following traumatic brain injury in pre-school children. *Brain Injury, 14*, 679–692.

Anderson, V., Morse, S., Catroppa, C., et al. (2004). Thirty month outcome from early childhood head injury: a prospective analysis of neurobehavioral recovery. *Brain, 127*, 2608–2620.

Cantu, R. (2001). Posttraumatic retrograde and anterograde amnesia: pathophysiology and implications in grading and safe return to play. *Journal of Athletic Training, 36*, 244–248.

Catroppa, C., & Anderson, V. (2003). Recovery and predictors of intellectual ability two years following paediatric traumatic brain injury. *Neuropsychological Rehabilitation, 13*, 517–536.

Catroppa, C., & Anderson, V. (2005). A prospective study of the recovery of attention from acute to 2 years following pediatric traumatic brain injury. *Journal of the International Neuropsychological Society, 11*, 84–98.

Centers for Disease Control and Prevention (2007) *Heads up: Brain injury in your practice. A tool kit for physicians.* Available via DIALOG. http://www.cdc.gov/concussion/HeadsUp/physicians_tool_kit.html of subordinate document. Cited 22 Feb 2011.

Centers for Disease Control and Prevention (2010). *What is traumatic brain injury?* Available via DIALOG. http://www.cdc.gov/traumaticbraininjury/statistics.html of subordinate document. Cited 22 Feb 2011.

Chapman, L., Wade, S., Walz, N., et al. (2010). Clinically significant behavior problems during the initial 18 months following early childhood traumatic brain injury. *Rehabilitation Psychology, 55*, 48–57.

Chapman, S., Ewing, C., & Mozzoni, M. (2005). Precision teaching and fluency training across cognitive, physical, and academic tasks in children with traumatic brain injury: a multiple baseline study. *Behavioral Interventions, 20*, 37–49.

Chevignard, M., Servant, V., Mariller, A., et al. (2009). Assessment of executive functioning in children after TBI with a naturalistic open-ended task: a pilot study. *Developmental Neurorehabilitation, 12*, 76–91.

Collins, M., Iverson, G., Lovell, M., et al. (2003). On-field predictors of neuropsychological and symptom deficit following sports-related concussion. *Clinical Journal of Sport Medicine, 13*, 222–229.

Collins, M., Lovell, M., & McKeag, D. (1999). Current issues in managing sports-related concussion. *Journal of the American Medical Association, 282*, 2388–2385.

Cole, W., Gerring, J., Gray, R., et al. (2008). Prevalence of aggressive behavior after severe paediatric traumatic brain injury. *Brain Injury, 22*, 932–939.

Conklin, H., Salorio, C., & Slomine, B. (2008). Working memory performance following paediatric traumatic brain injury. *Brain Injury, 22*, 847–857.

Fay, T., Yeates, K., Wade, S., et al. (2009). Predicting longitudinal patterns of functional deficits in children with traumatic brain injury. *Neuropsychology, 23*, 271–282.

Fenwick, T., & Anderson, V. (1999). Impairments of attention following childhood traumatic brain injury. *Child Neuropsychology, 5*, 213–223.

Gioia, G., Collins, M., & Isquith, P. (2008). Improving identification and diagnosis of mild TBI with evidence: Psychometric support for the Acute Concussion Evaluation (ACE). *The Journal of Head Trauma Rehabilitation, 23*, 230–242.

Gioia, G., Isquith, P., Schneider, J., et al. (2009). New approaches to assessment and monitoring of concussion in children. *Top Language Disorders, 29*, 266–281.

Gioia, G., Janusz, J., Isquith, P., et al. (2008). Psychometric properties of the parent and teacher Post-Concussion symptom Inventory (PCSI) for children and adolescents [Abstract]. *Journal of the International Neuropsychological Society, 14*(Suppl. 1), 204.

Hessen, E., Nestvold, K., & Anderson, V. (2007). Neuropsychological function 23 years after mild traumatic brain injury: a comparison of outcome after paediatric and adult head injuries. *Brain Injury, 21*, 963–979.

Horneman, G., & Emanuelson, I. (2009). Cognitive outcome in children and young adults who sustained severe and moderate traumatic brain injury 10 years earlier. *Brain Injury, 23*, 907–914.

Iverson, G. (2007). Predicting slow recovery from sport-related concussion: the new simple-complex distinction. *Clinical Journal of Sport Medicine, 17*, 31–37.

Iverson, G., Brooks, B., Collins, M., et al. (2006). Tracking neuropsychological recovery following concussion in sport. *Brain Injury, 20*, 245–252.

Kirkwood, M., Yeates, K., Taylor, H., et al. (2008). Management of pediatric mild traumatic brain injury: a neuropsychological review from injury through recovery. *The Clinical Neuropsychologist, 22*, 769–800.

Lau, B., Lovell, M., Collins, M., et al. (2009). Neurocognitive and symptom predictors of recovery in high school athletes. *Clinical Journal of Sport Medicine, 19*, 216–221.

Leblanc, N., Chen, S., Swank, P., et al. (2005). Response inhibition after traumatic brain injury (TBI) in children: impairment and recovery. *Developmental Neuropsychology, 28*, 829–848.

Levin, H., Song, J., Ewing-Cobbs, L., et al. (2001). Word fluency in relation to severity of closed head injury, associated frontal lesions, and age at injury in children. *Neuropsychologia, 39*, 122–131.

Lovell, M., Collins, M., Iverson, G., et al. (2003). Recovery from mild concussion in high school athletes. *Journal of Neurosurgery, 98*, 295–301.

Lovell M, Collins M, Maroon J (2002) ImPACT: The Best Approach to Concussion Management, User's Manual (Version 2.1) [computer software and manual]. ImPACT, Pittsburgh, PA.

Lovell, M., Iverson, G., Collins, M., et al. (2006). Measurement of symptoms following sport-related concussion: reliability and normative data for the Post-Concussion Scale. *Applied Neuropsychology, 13*, 166–174.

Mandalis, A., Kinsella, G., Ong, B., et al. (2007). Working memory and new learning following pediatric traumatic brain injury. *Developmental Neuropsychology, 32*, 683–701.

McCrea, M. (2008). *Mild traumatic brain injury and postconcussion syndrome*. New York: Oxford University Press.

McCrory, P., Meeuwisse, W., Johnston, K., et al. (2009). Consensus statement on concussion in sport: the 3rd international conference on concussion in sport held in Zurich, November 2008. *British Journal of Sports Medicine, 43*, 76–84.

Miller, L., & Donders, J. (2003). Prediction of educational outcome after pediatric traumatic brain injury. *Rehabilitation Psychology, 48*, 237–241.

Muscara, F., Catroppa, C., & Anderson, V. (2008). The impact of injury severity on executive function 7–10 years following pediatric traumatic brain injury. *Developmental Neuropsychology, 33*, 623–636.

Nadebaum, C., Anderson, V., & Catroppa, C. (2007). Executive function outcomes following traumatic brain injury in young children: a five year follow-up. *Developmental Neuropsychology, 32*, 703–728.

Park, B., Allen, D., Barney, S., et al. (2009). Structure of attention in children with traumatic brain injury. *Applied Neuropsychology, 16*, 1–10.

Slomine, B., Gerring, J., Grados, M., et al. (2002). Performance on measures of 'executive function' following pediatric traumatic brain injury. *Brain Injury, 16*, 759–772.

Sonnenberg, L., Dupuis, A., & Rumney, P. (2010). Pre-school traumatic brain injury and its impact on social development at 8 years of age. *Brain Injury, 24*, 1003–1007.

Taylor, H., Swartwout, M., Yeates, K., et al. (2008). Traumatic brain injury in young children: postacute effects on cognitive and social readiness skills. *Journal of the International Neuropsychological Society, 14*, 734–745.

Tsatsanis, K. (2005). Neuropsychological characteristics in autism and related conditions. In F. R. Volkmar, R. Paul, A. Klin, & D. Cohen (Eds.), *Handbook of autism and pervasive developmental disorders* (3rd ed.). Hoboken, NJ: Wiley.

Van Kampen, D., Lovell, M., Pardini, J., et al. (2006). The "value added" of neurocognitive testing after sports-related concussion. *The American Journal of Sports Medicine, 34,* 1–6.

Varni, J., Burwinkle, T., & Szer, I. (2004). The PedsQL multidimensional fatigue scale in pediatric rheumatology: reliability and validity. *The Journal of Rheumatology, 31,* 2494–2500.

Vriezen, E., & Pigott, S. (2002). The relationship between parental report on the BRIEF and performance-based measures of executive function in children with moderate to severe traumatic brain injury. *Child Neuropsychology, 8,* 296–303.

Wells, R., Minnes, P., & Phillips, M. (2009). Predicting social and functional outcomes for individuals sustaining paediatric traumatic brain injury. *Developmental Neurorehabilitation, 12,* 12–23.

Yeates, K., Armstrong, K., Janusz, J., et al. (2005). Long-term attention problems in children with traumatic brain injury. *Journal of the American Academy of Child and Adolescent Psychiatry, 44,* 574–584.

Yeates, K., Swift, E., Taylor, H., et al. (2004). Short- and long-term social outcomes following pediatric traumatic brain injury. *Journal of the International Neuropsychological Society, 10,* 412–426.

Part III
Additional Issues in Pediatric Concussion

Chapter 11
Premorbid Functional Considerations in Pediatric Concussion

Peter L. Stavinoha, Brianne Butcher, and Alice Ann Spurgin

11.1 Introduction

Clinicians working with children and adolescents with concussion and mild traumatic brain injury (TBI) can attest that substantial individual differences in functional outcomes exist even when injuries appear very similar. At least a portion of outcome variability seems accounted for by the interplay between injury characteristics (e.g., severity of injury) and noninjury-related factors. These noninjury characteristics include child-specific variables as well as environmental variables. After years of documenting outcomes from TBI in children, there is increasing interest in those factors that may moderate the negative impact of mild TBI in children, including greater awareness of the impact of the child's preinjury functioning and the potential to positively or negatively impact functional outcome following concussion.

This chapter focuses on preinjury variables that may influence neurocognitive and functional outcomes in individual children and adolescents following concussion. Specifically, research is reviewed on the influence of preinjury child characteristics (i.e., age, gender, cognitive and adaptive functioning, psychopathology, and genetic factors) and premorbid environmental characteristics (i.e., family psychosocial functioning, socioeconomic status [SES], race/ethnicity, and family environment) on injury expression. By better understanding the impact of these factors on outcome from concussion, clinicians will be better equipped to provide targeted guidance and intervention to hopefully improve outcome by managing risk factors that have the potential to complicate recovery from this common injury.

P.L. Stavinoha (✉) • A.A. Spurgin
Children's Medical Center of Dallas, University of Texas
Southwestern Medical Center, Dallas, TX, USA
e-mail: peter.stavinoha@childrens.com

B. Butcher
Children's Medical Center of Dallas, Dallas, TX, USA

J.N. Apps and K.D. Walter (eds.), *Pediatric and Adolescent Concussion:*
Diagnosis, Management and Outcomes, DOI 10.1007/978-0-387-89545-1_11,
© Springer Science+Business Media, LLC 2012

11.2 Preinjury Child Characteristics

11.2.1 Age

Research has shown variation in sequelae and recovery following brain injury in children related to age at time of injury. It is well accepted that insult to the brain at different stages in the developmental process can have distinct consequences for recovery and future learning (Kolb and Whishaw 2008). This research is supported by the understanding of critical periods of normal brain development and plasticity, as well as knowledge regarding the general biomechanics of concussion.

The current literature strongly suggests that the younger brain is more vulnerable to traumatic injury; however, much of the research excludes concussion or consolidates groups across TBI severity, which makes it difficult to draw firm conclusions regarding risk for complications associated with concussion. Younger children show greater potential for neural plasticity and potential for reorganization than more mature individuals. However, other factors related to diffuse injury including injury to brain systems responsible for new skill acquisition, smaller repertoire prior to injury creating a decreased "brain reserve," and a cascade of neurobiological consequences that prevent normal chemical and anatomic development have the potential to complicate outcomes from even mild TBI (Ewing-Cobbs et al. 2003; Kirkwood et al. 2006; Kolb and Whishaw 2008; Satz 1993).

Concussions involve rotational acceleration and/or deceleration forces that exert strain on neural tissue and vasculature (Barth et al. 2001; Kirkwood et al. 2006), and the effects of these forces may differ depending upon the age and developmental stage of the child given differences in the composition and neuronal organization of the brain. Age-dependent biological factors including skull geometry, suture elasticity, brain water content, cerebral blood volume, and level of myelination are also hypothesized to impact injury expression; however, the exact mechanisms are not currently clear (Kirkwood et al. 2006; Levin 2003; Prins and Hovda 2003).

While significant differences in outcomes based on age at time of injury have not consistently been found in school-age and adolescent populations, especially when severity of injury is restricted to mild TBI and concussion, traumatic brain injuries sustained in infancy or early childhood are associated with more persistent and severe deficits than those sustained later in life (Yeates et al. 2010). Greater risk for deficits include impairment in cognitive, academic, adaptive, social, and psychological domains of functioning (Anderson et al. 2004, 2009; Catroppa et al. 2007; Geraldina et al. 2003; Woodward et al. 1999; Wells et al. 2009).

When severity of brain injury was examined in relation to age, the age difference in outcome was only significant for severe and moderate TBI, with no significant discrepancy between outcomes based on age in the mild TBI groups (Anderson et al. 2009; Catroppa et al. 2007). This finding suggests that while young children are at increased risk for more severe and persisting functional deficits than older children and adolescents following brain injury, beneath a certain severity threshold, negative ramifications based on age appear to diminish. It is notable that the majority of studies on outcomes based on age have less than a 5-year follow-up period which has significant implications when making outcome predictions for individuals who sustain concussions at younger ages. Many cortical structures and neuronal pathways do not develop or fully myelinate until adolescence or early adulthood, thus deficits resulting from damage preventing normal development of these structures may be masked until later in adolescence or even young adulthood. Future research with populations that sustain concussions earlier in childhood should extend follow-up to assess long-term outcomes. Longitudinal follow-up over an extended period of time may clarify whether the severity threshold is a short-term phenomena or whether the effects of early concussion are present into adolescence and adulthood.

11.2.2   Gender

While it is well established that males – particularly young males – are at higher risk for acquiring a TBI (Mushkudiani et al. 2007), research regarding the effects of gender on pediatric mild TBI *outcomes* is sparse. Some studies have looked at gender as a predictor in more severe cases of TBI or in pediatric populations, but only a few studies on this topic have explicitly addressed pediatric TBI, and none has focused specifically on concussions and mild injuries. Thus, statements regarding the effects of gender on concussion and mild TBI in a pediatric population are tentative and inconclusive, being limited to extrapolation from studies of other populations or age groups.

One such study, conducted by Poggi et al. (2003), found that males aged 7–18 appear to be more at risk than females in that age range for social skills difficulties and emotional lability following a moderate to severe TBI. In an even broader sense, the study found that males at any age younger than 19 are at higher risk for socially maladaptive behaviors such as being withdrawn, passive, and closed-off in relationships following TBI. This indication that child and adolescent males with TBI are at greater risk than females for socialization difficulties may seem counter-intuitive given the greater risk for anxiety and depression in female TBI patients (Bay et al. 2009; Bell and Pepping 2001; Farace and Alves 2000; Glenn et al. 2001; Whelan-Goodinson et al. 2010). Nonetheless, Poggi et al. (2003) note that their sample of females younger than 19 years of age confirmed this trend, showing greater risk for anxiety and depression post-TBI compared to males. However, this did not translate to significant social skill difficulties or emotional lability, the key problems for males in the same age range.

There is also some evidence of differential neurocognitive outcomes following TBI based on gender. In a study focused on differences in outcome based on gender following sports-related concussions in high school and college athletes, females were found to exhibit a greater likelihood of cognitive impairment following concussion, and females also exhibited greater severity of neurocognitive impairment compared to males (Broshek et al. 2005). These authors concluded that these differences were not due to effects of injury severity, age, ethnicity, or baseline performance patterns, and they found that this gender difference persisted even after adjusting for the use of protective head gear.

In contrast, a preliminary study by Donders and Hoffman (2002) indicated that males ages 6–16 recovering from mild/moderate to severe TBI performed more poorly than females in that same age range on a verbal memory task as a function of increased retrieval deficits. Donders and Woodward (2003) then showed that boys ages 6–16 who sustained mild/moderate to severe TBI had more severe impairments in visual memory, verbal memory, and processing speed than age-matched girls, suggesting that gender moderates the effect of TBI severity on memory outcome. The authors suggested that processing speed deficits in their sample were responsible for the significantly worse performance on memory tasks by males as compared to females. This finding was confirmed in a broader study of mild to severe TBI patients aged 9–16, although in this study, gender was found to be an additive influence rather than a moderating variable – that is, it did not universally determine the relationship between injury variables and outcome (Donders and Nesbit-Greene 2004).

Adding to the mixed findings, a recent study suggested that adult females appear to retain better executive function following moderate to severe brain injury (Neimeier et al. 2007). At the same time, another study examining gender differences found males retain better visual analytic skills after mild to severe TBI, whereas females performed better in areas of working memory and language (Ratcliff et al. 2007).

Biological differences have emerged as a primary hypothesis for the occurrence of gender differences in TBI outcome, though this has not been studied specifically in the pediatric concussion population. While the relevance to concussion is not clear, gender-based anatomical outcome differences are evident in severe TBI. For example, studies of severe TBI suggest that females tend to have greater risk of brain swelling than males (Balestreri et al. 2003; Farin et al. 2003). Animal models suggest neurodegeneration following diffuse TBI is more rapid and severe in males than females (Kupina et al. 2003). If this holds true for humans, females may have a wider time frame during which interventions are maximally effective (Webbe 2006). A similarly designed animal study noted no impact of gender on neurodegeneration following focal TBI (Hall et al. 2005). The authors suggest that the more immediate anatomical effects of focal injuries may overwhelm any protective factors in females – namely, the effects of estrogen and progesterone which have been posited to protect against neural impairment following TBI (Bramlett and Dietrich 2001; Goss et al. 2003; Kupina et al. 2003; Ottochian et al. 2009; Wagner et al. 2004). However, the protective effect of female hormones following TBI is not a universal finding (Balestreri et al. 2003; Bruce-Keller et al. 2007; Davis et al. 2006; Farin et al. 2003).

While the studies described above suggest female gender may be a protective factor in outcome following TBI, Giza and Hovda (2001) have proposed that mild traumatic brain injuries may actually have worse effects in females due to female brains having higher cortical metabolic demands in the first place. They theorize that the decreased cerebral blood flow and increased glycemic demands following a mild TBI result in stronger and more prolonged symptoms in females. Indeed, females appear to be at greater risk for postconcussive syndrome (McCauley et al.

2001; Wood 2004) – that is, a set of physical, cognitive, emotional, or behavioral symptoms generally lasting more than 3 months following a mild TBI.

Ultimately, it is hard to make any definitive statements regarding the role of gender as either a risk or protective factor for the outcomes of mild TBI, and clearly this is an area that merits further investigation. Because the majority of research on gender differences has neither focused on children nor specifically examined concussion, hypotheses as to how these findings would extend to the pediatric concussion population are speculative. Further, it would be interesting to examine the possibility of an interaction between age and gender in studies of pediatric populations to determine whether the onset of puberty impacts gender differences following concussion and mild TBI.

11.2.3 Premorbid Cognitive Functioning

Brain reserve capacity (BRC) is a theoretical construct outlined by Satz (1993) which refers to the brain's capacity to cope with cerebral damage to minimize functional manifestations. According to the theory, once brain reserve is depleted beyond a critical threshold, specific clinical or functional deficits emerge or a significantly steeper decline in functioning commences. Common indices of BRC include intellectual abilities, learning and academic achievement, and adaptive functioning. In relation to pediatric concussions, preinjury BRC measured by premorbid intelligence, learning abilities, and adaptive skills may have significant implications for postconcussion recovery and functioning.

Children with preinjury learning problems including Attention Deficit/Hyperactivity Disorder (ADHD), Reading Disorders, Mathematics Disorder, and Learning Disorder-Not Otherwise Specified exhibit greater impairment in memory functioning, attention, executive functioning, adaptive behavior, and behavioral functioning compared to children without preexisting learning problems who sustain a TBI (Farmer et al. 2002; Ponsford et al. 1999; Sesma et al. 2008; Woodward et al. 1999). It is notable that study groups (TBI only vs. TBI with preexisting learning problems) did not differ by TBI severity; however, TBI severity within groups ranged from mild to severe, which impedes the application of these results specifically to the pediatric concussion population. In a small sample of children with moderate to severe TBI, Donders and Strom (1997) concluded that TBI can cause significant additional intellectual decline in children with preinjury learning disabilities compared to those children without a premorbid learning disability, though again the applicability to the pediatric concussion population is not entirely clear.

Similar to preinjury learning ability, level of adaptive functioning prior to injury is also associated with postinjury outcomes following TBI. Adaptive functioning involves skills necessary to interact effectively in society, make choices and judgments based on changing environmental demands, function safely and independently, and perform daily living skills necessary for self-care. Higher preinjury adaptive functioning predicts better recovery of intellectual abilities, language functions, and memory after mild to severe TBI (Anderson et al. 2004). Furthermore, school-age children with stronger preinjury adaptive functioning are less likely to demonstrate postinjury deficits in attention, hyperactivity, and impulsivity (Max et al. 2005).

Though research to date is sparse in pediatric populations regarding effects of developmental disabilities and mental retardation on functional outcomes after concussion, adult literature suggests that lower preinjury intellectual abilities are a risk factor for steeper cognitive declines after concussion in memory, verbal abilities, attention, and executive functioning (Johnstone et al. 1995). Additionally, adults with lower preinjury intellectual abilities generally demonstrate poorer emotional adjustment after head injury along with higher degrees of anxiety and depression (Wood and Rutterford 2006).

While these studies provide preliminary evidence supporting the "brain reserve threshold" in relation to TBI and level of cognitive and adaptive functioning prior to injury, future research is needed that specifically studies outcomes after pediatric concussion rather than combining groups across level of injury severity. Additionally, studies to date generally utilize parental report of preinjury learning problems and adaptive functioning rather than baseline neuropsychological data or other clearly objective evidence of performance. Recently, brief baseline neuropsychological screening has been advocated for and introduced in youth and high school sports programs as a model for best practice assessment in return to play issues after sports concussion (McCrory et al. 2005, 2009). This model may provide more sensitive and detailed evaluation of changes in cognitive functioning and learning after concussion.

Finally, more conclusive statements regarding functional outcomes and recommendations for targeted treatments could be provided if premorbid learning problems were separated into more specific groups (i.e., mental retardation, Reading Disorder, Mathematics Disorder, ADHD) rather than treated as a unitary construct. There is considerable variability in etiology and functioning between different learning disorders so implications for recovery after concussion may be very different depending upon the specific premorbid disorder.

11.2.4 Preinjury Psychopathology

Literature consistently demonstrates that TBI, even when mild in severity, is a significant risk factor for the development of anxiety, depression, and decreased psychological and social adjustment (Bay and Donders 2008; McCrory et al. 2009; Mooney and Speed 2001; Moore et al. 2006). The effects of preinjury psychopathology on recovery and outcome following TBI and concussion are less well established. In adult literature, preexisting depression has been found to negatively affect neurocognitive outcomes including intellectual functioning, verbal learning, verbal memory, processing speed, and executive functions following mild TBI (Cicerone and Kalmar 1997; Mooney and Speed 2001; Preece and Geffen 2007).

There is preliminary evidence that prior psychiatric illness increases risk for subsequent psychiatric disorders after mild TBI in children (Massagli et al. 2004). In this study, evidence of any new-onset psychiatric illness during the 3-year follow-up was estimated to occur in 26% of mild TBI subjects with no psychiatric history and in 55% of mild TBI subjects who had a prior psychiatric history. Increases in incidence of ADHD following mild TBI was the most significant contributor to postinjury psychiatric illness in this study. More research investigating effects of premorbid psychological disorders on postconcussion cognitive, psychological, and adaptive functioning is warranted in the pediatric population.

11.2.5   Genetic Factors

Genetic factors have been recently identified as playing a role in how the brain responds to injury (Jordan 2007), and this may have implications for outcomes following pediatric concussion. In adults, the apolipoprotein E allele 4 (APOE4) is associated with poorer outcomes from a variety of neurologic events including stroke and cardiopulmonary arrest, (Eichner et al. 2002; Strittmatter and Roses 1995) as well as earlier onset of Alzheimer's disease (Kim et al. 2009). Researchers have also linked possession of APOE4 to poorer broad functional outcomes from TBI in adults (Zhou et al. 2008), including association with poorer acute outcomes from mild TBI in adults (Liberman et al. 2002). These findings would certainly suggest that children possessing APOE4 may be at greater risk for poorer outcomes from milder brain injury.

However, only one study has examined the association between APOE4 and mild TBI in children (Moran et al. 2009). These researchers found that possession of APOE4 was associated with a poorer early functional response to mild TBI, though possession of the allele was not associated with differences in longer term neurocognitive outcome.

A number of additional genetic influences on outcome from TBI have been postulated (Jordan 2007), though thus far the findings are inconclusive and not of great relevance to the clinician working with children with concussion, as it is not typical for clinicians helping manage acute and postacute effects of concussion to have access to this information. Clearly genetic vulnerability and protective factors in mild TBI in children may be fruitful areas for additional study and may eventually lead to better understanding of relative risks as well as novel treatment for concussion and TBI in children.

11.3   Premorbid Environmental Characteristics

11.3.1   Family Factors

In considering the influence of home environment and family characteristics on pediatric TBI outcomes, several key factors emerge in the literature. Most prominently featured is the role of SES, often studied by looking at parental education level or occupation. Another factor that may impact outcome is ethnicity, which has been shown to have effects on pediatric TBI outcome independent of SES (Donders and Nesbit-Greene 2004). Finally, home environment, which includes a range of factors, from familial conflict to family stress/burden to parental psychiatric disorders may also play a role in moderating outcome from concussion and mild TBI. While research on the influences of many of these key factors on pediatric TBI outcomes has been extensive, studies specific to the concussion and mild TBI population are unfortunately lacking. However, certain trends are emerging that show promise for further research to isolate the impact of these factors on outcome from concussion in the pediatric population.

11.3.2 Socioeconomic Status

SES can be defined as the social position of an individual or family based on income, education level, and occupation. In attempting to explain the negative effects of low SES on child TBI outcome, one theory is that these families have limited access to resources in the community that could improve the child's prognosis. Another leading hypothesis is that low SES parents face other difficulties and stressors that limit their personal resources – financially, socially, and psychologically – for assisting the child's recovery (Max et al. 2005; Sesma et al. 2008; Taylor et al. 2002). In some ways, this mimics the BRC hypothesis by suggesting that "family resource reserve" is of notable importance in determining outcome from TBI.

In a study of both SES and home environment factors, Taylor et al. (2002) found that a composite index of SES, years of maternal education, and family income was the factor most consistently associated with outcome from moderate and severe TBI in children. Higher scores on that composite index, indicating higher SES and family variables, predicted better outcomes. Lower SES has been associated with more behavioral problems, poorer academic outcomes, and slower development of social skills in children following TBI (Max et al. 2005; Schwartz et al. 2003; Sesma et al. 2008; Taylor et al. 2002; Yeates et al. 2004). Interestingly, evidence regarding cognitive outcomes of multiple mild TBIs in children (Bijur et al. 1996) suggests that SES may play a larger role than biological aspects of injury in predicting long-term cognitive outcomes of mild TBI in childhood.

Among variables thought to comprise SES, findings appear less significant for parental education level. Luis and Mittenberg (2002) studied a full range of mild to severe TBI children and concluded that parental education level did not predict the development of mood or anxiety disorders in these children postinjury. Similarly, neither parental education nor household income was related to social or functional outcomes of children in a sample of predominantly mild TBI (Wells et al. 2009). However, parental occupation has been found to be associated with intellectual, language, and memory outcomes in children with mild to severe TBI (Anderson et al. 2004). Thus, while findings regarding the effect of SES are fairly congruent, studies that break down the factors that comprise SES show less consistent results. More research is clearly needed to delineate the relative risk and protection of these factors in cases of pediatric concussion.

11.3.3   Race and Ethnicity

It is important to note that race and ethnicity, independent of SES, also have been shown to play a role in predicting brain injury outcomes. In adult populations, some evidence suggests that ethnic minorities – specifically, African Americans and Hispanics – have worse long-term functional outcomes and quality of life following TBI (Arango-Lasprilla et al. 2009, 2007a, b; Staudenmayer et al. 2007). In pediatric populations, evidence is not consistent. Some studies suggest that there are no ethnicity-related differences in mortality, medical disposition, or functional outcomes in children with mild to severe TBI (Bedell 2008; Howard et al. 2005; Lopez et al. 2006). Others contradict this assertion, presenting evidence that African American children have worse outcomes in terms of both mortality and adaptive functioning (Falcone et al. 2008; Haider et al. 2007; Martin et al. 2010). Specifically, Haider and colleagues found that Hispanic and Caucasian children with moderate to severe TBI had comparable outcomes, but African American children had worse clinical and functional outcomes. Because targeted support and education may moderate the impact of ethnicity on outcome from mild TBI, more research is needed on this topic to better inform clinicians managing these injuries in children.

11.3.4   Family Environment

Family environment is another key factor in determining outcome of pediatric TBI – in fact, there is some indication that family environment may be a stronger moderator of outcomes than SES (Ewing-Cobbs et al. 2004; Max et al. 2005; Yeates et al. 1997) and even injury severity (Rivara et al. 1996). In general, higher levels of family burden, parental psychological distress, and family conflict/dysfunction are associated with a broad range of poorer outcomes for children with TBI, often even after controlling for SES and ethnicity (Kirkwood et al. 2008; Ponsford et al. 1999; Rivara et al. 1996; Sesma et al. 2008; Taylor et al. 1999, 2002; Wells et al. 2009; Yeates et al. 1997, 2004). While family environment and race/ethnicity have independent effects on outcome after TBI, there can be interactions between these variables as well. Race/ethnicity serves as a factor in creating the family environment, as Yeates et al. (2002) found that, independent of SES, race was related to the type of coping strategies utilized by families following TBI with Caucasian families tending to have more effective belief systems surrounding recovery from injury than African American families.

A consistent finding across many studies is that the family environment influences a child's post-TBI behavioral and functional outcomes more than cognitive outcomes (Yeates 2010). For example, Yeates et al. (1997) found that family environment accounted for up to 25% of the variance in the child's outcome in adaptive functioning but no more than 10% of the variance in cognitive outcomes. However, this is not a universal finding, as Catroppa et al. (2008) found no significant association between measures of family conflict and intimacy and child TBI outcome.

There are several hypotheses regarding the influence of the family environment on pediatric TBI outcomes. One is that the physiological and neurobehavioral effects of TBI reduce a child's functional independence, making the child more susceptible to a family environment that provides less psychological and functional support (Taylor et al. 1999). Another is that a strong family environment may actively facilitate the child's recovery on a neurological level (Max et al. 2005; Taylor et al. 1999, 2002), a hypothesis that is supported by animal research (Kolb 1989). The inverse suggests that when a strong, adaptive family environment is absent, neurological recovery may be reduced, a mechanism by which parental psychiatric issues and maladaptive coping styles can negatively impact the child's outcome (Max et al. 2005).

Finally, when considering the impact of family factors on pediatric TBI outcome, there is a vicious cycle that must be taken into account – that is, at the same time the family environment can impact outcome from TBI, having a child with TBI can negatively impact long-term family functioning following the injury (Ponsford and Schonberger 2010; Rivara et al. 1996; Schwartz et al. 2003; Wade et al. 2006; Yeates et al. 1997). Key factors that appear to moderate the impact of pediatric TBI on caregivers include SES, race/ethnicity, preinjury family functioning, resources (particularly social support), presence of other family stressors, and the severity of the injury (Rivara et al. 1996; Wade et al. 2005; Wade et al. 2006). Many of these factors interact; for example, the combination of a severe injury and low SES tends to result in higher levels of parental stress (Wade et al. 2006).

The vicious cycle – wherein pediatric TBI can negatively impact the family environment, which then negatively impacts the child's outcome – is illustrated by findings that with increasing years postinjury, parental distress and family dysfunction increase (Rivara et al. 1996; Wade et al. 2006). This vicious cycle is a phenomenon that, like all the family factors mentioned in this section, deserves further research in the concussion and mild TBI population, particularly as it has been documented only in moderate to severe TBI children to this point and has not been thoroughly examined following milder levels of TBI.

11.4 Summary

While research regarding cognitive outcomes from concussion and mild TBI in children is not consistent, these children do appear to experience greater levels of postconcussive emotional, behavioral, somatic, and cognitive difficulties compared to children with injuries that did not involve the head (Yeates 2010). As discussed above, there are a number of noninjury-related factors that may play a role in affecting outcome from concussion, including factors associated with increased risk for poor outcome as well as factors that are potentially protective to the child who has experienced concussion. Given that the vast majority of research on these noninjury factors has involved mixed TBI populations or has focused on moderate and severe injuries, the impact of factors such as age, gender, genetic factors, preinjury functioning and psychopathology, and a variety of socioeconomic and family characteristics is not entirely clear. Studies of more severe TBI in children as well as the adult TBI literature suggest that these factors may all have a role in outcome following concussion in children, but clearly more research is needed to clarify interactions and contributions of these variables to outcome from concussion in a pediatric population. Further clarification of these issues is imperative to better inform clinicians working with these children and families regarding the most appropriate intervention and guidance specific to identifiable risk and protective factors that are unique to that child and family.

11.5 Key Points

Age. In more severe traumatic brain injuries, earlier age has been associated with poorer outcome, though conclusive statements regarding the impact of age on concussion outcome cannot be made.

Gender. Similar to age, there is some literature, though not particularly consistent or cohesive, suggesting gender differences in outcomes from moderate and severe TBI, with the implication that there may be differences in outcome based on gender following pediatric concussion.

Premorbid Cognitive Functioning. In general, learning and cognitive difficulties prior to TBI are associated with poorer outcome.

Preinjury Psychopathology. Evidence suggests that children with preexisting psychiatric difficulties are at risk for poorer outcome following TBI.

SES. Studies of outcomes from TBI have demonstrated that lower SES tends to be associated with worse functional outcome, presumably because fewer family resources are available to moderate the effects of TBI.

Race and Ethnicity. Race and ethnicity, independent of SES, also have been shown to play a role in predicting brain injury outcomes, with some studies suggesting ethnic minorities are at greater risk for poorer outcomes from TBI, though the finding is not universal.

Family Environment. Higher levels of family burden, parental psychological distress, and family conflict/dysfunction are associated with a broad range of poorer outcomes for children across TBI severity.

Further Research. Research specifically investigating risk and protective factors associated with outcome from pediatric concussion is lacking. The TBI literature in general provides some guidance, but each of the factors discussed in this chapter requires additional study.

References

Anderson, V., Morse, S., Catroppa, C., Haritou, F., & Rosenfeld, J. (2004). Thirty month outcome from early childhood head injury: a prospective analysis of neurobehavioral recovery. *Brain, 127,* 2608–2620.

Anderson, V., Catroppa, C., Morse, S., Haritou, F., & Rosenfeld, J. (2009). Intellectual outcome from preschool traumatic brain injury: a 5-year prospective, longitudinal study. *Pediatrics, 124,* 1064–1071.

Arango-Lasprilla, J., Rosenthal, M., Deluca, J., Cifu, D., Hanks, R., & Komaroff, E. (2007). Functional outcomes from inpatient rehabilitation after traumatic brain injury: how do hispanics fare? *Archives of Physical Medicine and Rehabilitation, 88*(1), 11–8.

Arango-Lasprilla, J., Rosenthal, M., Deluca, J., Komaroff, E., Sherer, M., Cifu, D., et al. (2007). Traumatic brain injury and functional outcomes: does minority status matter? *Brain Injury, 21*(7), 701–708.

Arango-Lasprilla, J., Ketchum, J., Gary, K., Hart, T., Corrigan, J., Forster, L., et al. (2009). Race/ethnicity differences in satisfaction with life among persons with traumatic brain injury. *NeuroRehabilitation, 24*(1), 5–14.

Balestreri, M., Steiner, L., & Czosnyka, M. (2003). Sex related differences and traumatic brain injury. *Journal of Neurosurgery, 99,* 616.

Barth, J., Freeman, J., Broshek, D., & Varney, R. (2001). Acceleration-deceleration sport-related concussion: the gravity of it all. *Journal of Athletic Training, 36,* 253–256.

Bay, E., & Donders, J. (2008). Risk factors for depressive symptoms after mild-to-moderate traumatic brain injury. *Brain Injury, 22*(3), 233–241.

Bay, E., Sikorskii, A., & Saint-Arnault, D. (2009). Sex differences in depressive symptoms and their correlates after mild-to-moderate traumatic brain injury. *Journal of Neurosurgical Nursing, 41*(6), 298–309.

Bedell, G. (2008). Functional outcomes of school-age children with acquired brain injuries at discharge from inpatient rehabilitation. *Brain Injury, 22*(4), 313–324.

Bell, K., & Pepping, M. (2001). Women and traumatic brain injury. *Physical Medicine and Rehabilitation Clinics of North America, 12,* 169–182.

Bijur, P., Haslum, M., & Golding, J. (1996). Cognitive outcomes of multiple mild head injuries in children. *Journal of Developmental and Behavioral Pediatrics, 17,* 143–148.

Bramlett, H., & Dietrich, W. (2001). Neuropathological protection after traumatic brain injury in intact female rats versus males or ovariectomized females. *Journal of Neurotrauma, 18,* 891–900.

Broshek, D., Kaushik, T., Freeman, J., Erlanger, D., Webbe, F., & Barth, J. (2005). Gender differences in outcome from sports-related concussion. *Journal of Neurosurgery, 102,* 856–863.

Bruce-Keller, A., Dimayuga, F., Reed, J., Wang, C., Angers, R., Wilson, M., et al. (2007). Gender and estrogen manipulation do not affect traumatic brain injury in mice. *Journal of Neurotrauma, 24*(1), 203–215.

Catroppa, C., Anderson, V., Morse, S., Haritou, F., & Rosenfeld, V. (2007). Children's attentional skills 5 years post-TBI. *Journal of Pediatric Psychology, 32*(3), 354–369.

Catroppa, C., Anderson, V., Morse, S., Haritou, F., & Rosenfeld, J. (2008). *Journal of Pediatric Psychology, 33*(7), 707–718.

Cicerone, K., & Kalmar, K. (1997). Does premorbid depression influence post-concussive symptoms and neuropsychological functioning? *Brain Injury, 11,* 643–648.

Davis, D., Douglas, D., Smith, W., Sise, M., Vilke, G., Holbrook, T., et al. (2006). Traumatic brain injury outcomes in pre- and post-menopausal females versus age-matched males. *Journal of Neurotrauma, 23*(2), 140–148.

Donders, J., & Hoffman, N. (2002). Gender differences in learning and memory after pediatric traumatic brain injury. *Neuropsychology, 16*(4), 491–499.

Donders, J., & Nesbit-Greene, K. (2004). Predictors of neuropsychological test performance after pediatric traumatic brain injury. *Assessment, 11*(4), 275–284.

Donders, J., & Strom, D. (1997). The effects of traumatic brain injury on children with learning disability. *Pediatric Rehabilitation, 1*(3), 179–184.

Donders, J., & Woodward, H. (2003). Gender as a moderator of memory after traumatic brain injury in children. *The Journal of Head Trauma Rehabilitation, 18*, 106–115.

Eichner, J., Dunn, S., Perveen, G., Thompson, D., Stewart, K., & Stroehla, B. (2002). Apolipoprotein E polymorphism and cardiovascular disease: a HuGE review. *American Journal of Epidemiology, 155*(6), 487–495.

Ewing-Cobbs, L., Barnes, M., & Fletcher, J. (2003). Early brain injury in children: development and reorganization of cognitive function. *Developmental Neuropsychology, 24*, 669–704.

Ewing-Cobbs, L., Barnes, M., Fletcher, J., Levin, H., Swank, P., & Song, J. (2004). Modeling of longitudinal academic achievement scores after pediatric traumatic brain injury. *Developmental Neuropsychology, 25*(1&2), 107–133.

Falcone, R., Jr., Martin, C., Brown, R., & Garcia, V. (2008). Despite overall low pediatric head injury mortality, disparities exist between races. *Journal of Pediatric Surgery, 43*(10), 1858–1864.

Farace, E., & Alves, W. (2000). Do women fare worse: a metaanalysis of gender differences in traumatic brain injury outcome. *Journal of Neurosurgery, 93*, 539–545.

Farin, A., Deutsch, R., Biegon, A., & Marshal, L. (2003). Sex-related differences in patients with severe head injury: greater susceptibility to brain swelling in female patients 50 years of age and younger. *Journal of Neurosurgery, 98*, 32–36.

Farmer, J., Kanne, S., Haut, J., Williams, J., Johnstone, B., & Kirk, K. (2002). Memory functioning following traumatic brain injury in children with premorbid learning problems. *Developmental Neuropsychology, 22*(2), 455–469.

Geraldina, P., Mariarosaria, L., Annarita, A., Susanna, G., Michela, S., Alessandro, D., et al. (2003). Neuropsychiatric sequelae in TBI: a comparison across different age groups. *Brain Injury, 17*(10), 835–846.

Giza, C., & Hovda, D. (2001). The neurometabolic cascade of concussion. *Journal of Athletic Training, 36*, 228–235.

Glenn, M., O'Neil- Pirozzi, T., Goldstein, R., et al. (2001). Depression amongst outpatients with traumatic brain injury. *Brain Injury, 15*, 811–818.

Goss, C., Hoffman, S., & Stein, D. (2003). Behavioral effects and anatomic correlates after brain injury: a progesterone dose-response study. *Pharmacology Biochemistry and Behavior, 76*, 231–242.

Haider, A., Efron, D., Haut, E., DiRusso, S., Sullivan, T., & Cornwell, E. (2007). Black children experience worse clinical and functional outcomes after traumatic brain injury: an analysis of the National Pediatric Trauma Registry. *The Journal of Trauma, 62*(5), 1259–1263.

Hall, E., Gibson, T., & Pavel, K. (2005). Lack of a gender difference in post-traumatic neurodegeneration in the mouse controlled cortical impact injury model. *Journal of Neurotrauma, 22*(6), 669–679.

Howard, I., Joseph, J., & Natale, J. (2005). Pediatric traumatic brain injury: do racial/ethnic disparities exist in brain injury severity, mortality, or medical disposition? *Ethnicity & Disease, 15*(4 Suppl 5), 51–56.

Johnstone, B., Hexum, B., & Ashkahazi, G. (1995). Extent of cognitive decline in traumatic brain injury based on estimates of premorbid intelligence. *Brain Injury, 9*(4), 377–384.

Jordan, B. (2007). Genetic influences on outcome following traumatic brain injury. *Neurochemical Research, 32*, 905–915.

Kim, J., Basak, J., & Holtzman, D. (2009). The role of apolipoprotein E in Alzheimer's disease. *Neuron, 63*(3), 287–303.

Kirkwood, M., Yeates, K., & Wilson, P. (2006). Pediatric sport-related concussion: a review of the clinical management of an oft-neglected population. *Pediatrics, 117*(4), 1359–1371.

Kirkwood, M., Yeates, K., Taylor, H., Randolph, C., McCrea, M., & Anderson, V. (2008). Management of mild pediatric traumatic brain injury: a neuropsychological review from injury through recovery. *Clinical Neuropsychology, 22*(5), 769–800.

Kolb, B. (1989). Brain development, plasticity, and behavior. *The American Psychologist, 44*, 1203–1212.

Kolb, B., & Whishaw, I. (2008). *Fundamentals of human neuropsychology* (6th ed.). New York: Worth Publishers.

Kupina, N., Detloff, M., Bobrowski, W., Snyder, B., & Hall, E. (2003). Cytoskeletal protein degradation and neurodegeneration evolves differently in males and females following experimental head injury. *Experimental Neurology, 180*, 55–72.

Levin, H. (2003). Neuroplasticity following non-penetrating traumatic brain injury. *Brain Injury, 17*, 665–674.

Liberman, J., Stewart, W., Wesnes, K., & Troncoso, J. (2002). Apolipoprotein E ε4 and short-term recovery from predominantly mild brain injury. *Neurology, 58*, 1038–1044.

Lopez, A., Tilford, J., Anand, K., Jo, C., Green, J., Aitken, M., et al. (2006). Variation in pediatric intensive care therapies and outcomes by race, gender, and insurance status. *Pediatric Critical Care Medicine, 7*(1), 2–6.

Luis, C., & Mittenberg, W. (2002). Mood and anxiety disorders following pediatric traumatic brain injury: a prospective study. *Journal of Clinical and Experimental Neuropsychology, 24*(3), 270–279.

Martin, C., Care, M., Rangel, E., Brown, R., Garcia, V., & Falcone, R., Jr. (2010). Severity of head computed tomography scan findings fail to explain racial differences in mortality following child abuse. *American Journal of Surgery, 199*(2), 210–215.

Massagli, T., Fann, J., Burington, B., Jaffe, K., Katon, W., & Thompson, R. (2004). Psychiatric illness after mild traumatic brain injury in children. *Archives of Physical Medicine and Rehabilitation, 85*, 1428–1434.

Max, J., Schachar, R., Levin, H., Ewing-Cobbs, L., Chapman, S., Dennis, M., et al. (2005). Predictors of secondary attention-deficit/hyperactivity disorder in children and adolescents 6 to 24 months after traumatic brain injury. *Journal of the American Academy of Child and Adolescent Psychiatry, 44*(10), 1041–1049.

McCauley, S., Boake, C., Levin, H., Contant, C., & Song, J. (2001). Post-concussional disorder following mild to moderate traumatic brain injury: anxiety, depression, and social support as risk factors and co-morbidities. *Journal of Clinical and Experimental Neuropsychology, 23*(6), 792–808.

McCrory, P., Johnston, K., Meeuwisse, W., Aubry, M., Cantu, R., Dvorak, J., et al. (2005). Summary and agreement statement of the 2nd International Conference on Concussion in Sport, Prague 2004. *Clinical Journal of Sport Medicine, 15*, 48–55.

McCrory, P., Meeuwisse, W., Johnston, K., Dvorak, J., Aubry, M., Molloy, M., et al. (2009). Consensus statement on concussion in sport, 3 rd International Conference on Concussion in Sport Held in Zurich, November 2008. *Clinical Journal of Sport Medicine, 19*, 185–200.

Mooney, G., & Speed, J. (2001). The association between mild traumatic brain injury and psychiatric conditions. *Brain Injury, 15*, 865–877.

Moore, E., Terryberry-Spohr, L., & Hope, D. (2006). Mild traumatic brain injury and anxiety sequelae: a review of the literature. *Brain Injury, 20*(2), 117–132.

Moran, L., Taylor, H., Ganesalingam, K., Gastier-Foster, J., Frick, J., Bangert, B., et al. (2009). Apolipoprotein E4 as a predictor of outcomes in pediatric mild traumatic brain injury. *Journal of Neurotrauma, 26*, 1489–1495.

Mushkudiani, N., Engel, D., Steyerberg, E., Butcher, I., Lu, J., Marmarou, A., et al. (2007). Prognostic value of demographic characteristics in traumatic brain injury: results from the IMPACT study. *Journal of Neurotrauma, 24*, 259–269.

Neimeier, J., Marwitz, J., Lesher, K., Walker, W., & Bushnik, T. (2007). Gender differences in executive functions following traumatic brain injury. *Neuropsychological Rehabilitation, 17*(3), 293–313.

Ottochian, M., Salim, A., Berry, C., Chan, L., Wilson, M., & Marguiles, D. (2009). Severe traumatic brain injury: is there a gender difference in mortality? *American Journal of Surgery, 197*(2), 155–158.

Poggi, G., Liscio, M., Adduci, A., Galiati, S., Sommovigo, M., Degrate, A., et al. (2003). Neuropsychiatric sequelae in TBI: a comparison across different age groups. *Brain Injury, 17*(10), 835–846.

Ponsford, J., & Schonberger, M. (2010). Family functioning and emotional state two and five years after traumatic brain injury. *Journal of the International Neuropsychological Society, 16*, 306–317.

Ponsford, J., Willmott, C., Rothwell, A., Cameron, P., Ayton, G., Nelms, R., et al. (1999). Cognitive and behavioral outcome following mild traumatic head injury in children. *The Journal of Head Trauma Rehabilitation, 14*(4), 360–372.

Preece, M., & Geffen, G. (2007). The contribution of pre-existing depression to the acute cognitive sequelae of mild traumatic brain injury. *Brain Injury, 21*(9), 951–961.

Prins, M., & Hovda, D. (2003). Developing experimental models to address traumatic brain injury in children. *Journal of Neurotrauma, 20*, 123–137.

Ratcliff, J., Greenspan, A., Goldstein, F., Stringer, A., Bushnik, T., Hammond, F., et al. (2007). Gender and traumatic brain injury: do the sexes fare differently? *Brain Injury, 21*(10), 1023–1030.

Rivara, J., Jaffe, K., Polissar, N., Fay, G., Liao, S., & Martin, K. (1996). Predictors of family functioning and change 3 years after traumatic brain injury in children. *Archives of Physical Medicine and Rehabilitation, 77*, 754–764.

Satz, P. (1993). Brain reserve capacity on symptom onset after brain injury: a formulation and review of evidence for threshold theory. *Neuropsychology, 7*(3), 273–295.

Schwartz, L., Taylor, H., Drotar, D., Yeates, K., Wade, S., & Stancin, T. (2003). Long-term behavior problems following pediatric traumatic brain injury: prevalence, predictors, and correlates. *Journal of Pediatric Psychology, 28*(4), 251–263.

Sesma, H., Slomine, B., Ding, R., McCarthy, M., & The Children's Health After Trauma (CHAT) Study Group. (2008). Executive functioning in the first year after pediatric traumatic brain injury. *Pediatrics, 121*, 1686–1695.

Staudenmayer, K., Diaz-Arrastia, R., de Oliveira, A., Gentilello, L., & Shafi, S. (2007). Ethnic disparities in long-term functional outcomes after traumatic brain injury. *The Journal of Trauma, 63*(6), 1364–1369.

Strittmatter, W., & Roses, A. (1995). Apolipoportein E and Alzheimer disease. *Proceedings of the National Academy of Sciences of the United States of America, 92*, 4725–4727.

Taylor, H., Yeates, K., Wade, S., Drotar, D., Klein, S., & Stancin, T. (1999). Influences on first-year recovery from traumatic brain injury in children. *Neuropsychology, 13*, 76–89.

Taylor, H., Yeates, K., Wade, S., Drotar, D., Stancin, T., & Minich, N. (2002). A prospective study of long- and short-term outcomes after traumatic brain injury in children: behavior and achievement. *Neuropsychology, 16*, 15–27.

Wade, S., Wolfe, C., Brown, T., & Pestian, J. (2005). Putting the pieces together: preliminary efficacy of a web-based family intervention for children with traumatic brain injury. *Journal of Pediatric Psychology, 30*, 437–442.

Wade, S., Taylor, H., Yeates, K., Drotar, D., Stancin, T., Minich, N., et al. (2006). Long-term parental and family adaptation following pediatric brain injury. *Journal of Pediatric Psychology, 10*, 1072–1083.

Wagner, A., Bayir, H., Ren, D., Puccio, A., Zafonte, R., & Kochanek, P. (2004). Relationships between cerebrospinal fluid markers of excitotoxicity, ischemia, and oxidative damage after severe TBI: the impact of gender, age, and hypothermia. *Journal of Neurotrauma, 21*(2), 125–136.

Webbe, F. (2006). Definition, physiology, and severity of cerebral concussion. In R. J. Echemendia (Ed.), *Sports neuropsychology: assessment and management of traumatic brain injury* (pp. 45–70). New York: The Guilford Press.

Wells, R., Minnes, P., & Phillips, M. (2009). Predicting social and functional outcomes for individuals sustaining paediatric traumatic brain injury. *Developmental Neurorehabilitation, 12*(1), 12–23.

Whelan-Goodinson, R., Ponsford, J., Schonberger, M., & Johnston, L. (2010). Predictors of psychiatric disorders following traumatic brain injury. *The Journal of Head Trauma Rehabilitation, 25*, 320–329.

Wood, R. (2004). Understanding the 'miserable minority': a diathesis-stress paradigm for post-concussional syndrome. *Brain Injury, 18*(11), 1135–1153.

Wood, R., & Rutterford, N. (2006). The impact of mild developmental learning difficulties on neuropsychological recovery from head trauma. *Brain Injury, 20*(5), 477–484.

Woodward, H., Winterhalther, K., Donders, J., Hackbarth, R., Kuldanek, A., & Sanfilippo, D. (1999). Prediction of neurobehavioral outcome 1–5 years post pediatric traumatic head injury. *The Journal of Head Trauma Rehabilitation, 14*(4), 351–359.

Yeates, K. (2010). Traumatic brain injury. In K. Yeates, M. Ris, H. Taylor, & B. Pennington (Eds.), *Pediatric neuropsychology, research theory, and practice* (2nd ed., pp. 112–146). New York: The Guilford Press.

Yeates, K., Taylor, H., Drotar, D., Wade, S., Klein, S., Stancin, T., et al. (1997). Preinjury family environment as a determinant of recovery from traumatic brain injuries in school-age children. *Journal of the International Neuropsychological Society, 3*, 617–630.

Yeates, K., Taylor, G., Woodrome, S., Wade, S., Stancin, T., & Drotar, D. (2002). Race as a moderator of parent and family outcomes following pediatric traumatic brain injury. *Journal of Pediatric Psychology, 27*(4), 393–403.

Yeates, K., Swift, E., Taylor, H., Wade, S., Drotar, D., Stancin, T., et al. (2004). Short- and long-term social outcomes following pediatric traumatic brain injury. *Journal of the International Neuropsychological Society, 10*, 412–426.

Zhou, W., Xu, D., Peng, X., Zhang, Q., Jia, J., & Crutcher, K. (2008). Meta-analysis of APOE4 allele and outcome after traumatic brain injury. *Journal of Neurotrauma, 25*(4), 279–290.

Chapter 12
Developmental Considerations in Pediatric Concussion Evaluation and Management

Gerard A. Gioia, Christopher G. Vaughan, and Maegan D.S. Sady

12.1 Introduction

Evaluation and management of concussion in children and adolescents present a number of unique issues for the clinician. Regardless of age at injury, the primary tasks of the concussion evaluation are to identify postconcussion signs and symptoms relative to preinjury status, and to delineate the impact of the ongoing, changing symptoms on the individual's everyday life. The primary purpose of concussion treatment and management is then to arrange the proper environmental conditions to allow expeditious resolution of the presenting symptoms. While the key areas for clinical assessment of children with concussion are generally similar to those of adults (i.e., postconcussion symptoms, specific neuropsychological functions), there are important differences in the approach to assessment and management due to differences in maturational level of cognitive and emotional functioning, environmental

G.A. Gioia(✉)
Division of Pediatric Neuropsychology, Director Safe Concussion Outcome Recovery and Education (SCORE) Program

Associate Professor, Departments of Pediatric and Psychiatry and Behavioral Sciences, George Washington University of Medicine, Washington, DC, USA
e-mail: ggioia@childrensnational.org

C.G. Vaughan
Division of Pediatric Neuropsychology, Children's National Medical Center

Assistant Professor, Departments of Pediatrics and Psychiatry and Behavioral Sciences, George Washington University School of Medicine, Washington, DC, USA

M.D.S. Sady
Division of Pediatric Neuropsychology,
Children's National Medical Center, Washington, DC, USA

J.N. Apps and K.D. Walter (eds.), *Pediatric and Adolescent Concussion:*   151
Diagnosis, Management and Outcomes, DOI 10.1007/978-0-387-89545-1_12,
© Springer Science+Business Media, LLC 2012

demands, and neural development. For these reasons, pediatric concussion evaluation is not a simple "downsizing" or application of an adult assessment model to children. While the extant adult-oriented concussion evaluation tools have provided a reasonable starting point, they ultimately require significant modifications from a developmental perspective for use with children and adolescents. Such modifications should account for differences in neurocognitive development and differences in the child's ability to detect and report symptoms and changes from pre- to postconcussion. To frame the pediatric concussion evaluation, the evaluation of children at different ages requires an approach that is sensitive to developmental differences in injury manifestation and recovery, and to developmental differences in the child's capacity to engage actively in the evaluation and treatment process (Varni et al. 2007a, b). Thus, parents and often other key adults such as teachers and coaches will play an important complementary role in the evaluation and treatment process, particularly in the younger child, but also in the adolescent (De Los Reyes and Kazdin 2005; Varni et al. 2007a, b).

We present a model for clinical evaluation and management of concussion in children and adolescents at the acute and postacute stages that incorporates multiple methods and informants and that is guided by the specific goals and timing of the service in relation to the injury. Pediatric concussion evaluation at the postacute stage requires a detailed assessment of the injury characteristics and history (including preinjury risk factors), in combination with current neurocognitive, symptom, and social–emotional status, all with consideration of change from preinjury (baseline) function. We advocate a standardized assessment approach using methods that tap multiple domains of the child's functioning and gather input from key informants across settings. The combination of structured symptom rating scales and neuropsychological testing with a well-defined understanding of the injury within the context of the child's developmental, medical, and educational history provides a comprehensive view of the injury's effects and impact in the child's everyday world.

12.1.1 *Developmental Considerations*

The capacity of the child to be an active participant in the concussion evaluation and management must be considered for each individual case. The child's age and ability to participate determines which assessment tools are developmentally appropriate. A review of the available clinical tools commonly used for assessing concussion reveals differences across the age spectrum in the availability of developmentally appropriate measures, in the reliability of measures, and in the format of measures (Gioia et al. 2009b). Few standardized tools exist to meet the needs of the preadolescent pediatric population, especially with respect to serial assessment (Gioia et al. 2009b; Kirkwood et al. 2006; Lovell and Fazio 2008). Furthermore, younger children differ from adolescents in their capacity to adhere independently to treatment recommendations (e.g., ability to take self-imposed breaks to avoid overexertion), requiring a developmentally appropriate framework for intervention. At a more fundamental level, there is emerging evidence from animal studies with some associated evidence from human research that the effects of concussive forces to the brain may differ depending on age or developmental maturity (Giza and Prins 2006). Thus, the complex interaction between the developing brain and the child's situational and developmental characteristics can result in a unique manifestation of the injury and treatment approach for any particular individual.

A comprehensive, developmentally sensitive, model of concussion evaluation requires four key elements: (1) an understanding of typical development and developmentally appropriate behavior, (2) developmentally appropriate measures of the injury's clinical manifestations, (3) involvement of additional key persons who are familiar with the child in the assessment process, and (4) expectation that recovery may be longer in the younger child (Field et al. 2003; Moser et al. 2005; Pellman et al. 2006; McKinlay et al. 2002).

While some may view children as "little adults," developmentally sensitive practitioners know full well that children's brain and cognitive development are individualized and interact with the environment in unique ways, requiring care providers to view the concussion from a developmental, "child-world," perspective (Bernstein and Waber 1990). Understanding an injury to a 5-year-old who collides with another player in a soccer game is different from a 15-year-old skateboarder who falls backward onto concrete in a half-pipe. In each of these youngsters, there is developmental variability in cognitive development, in expression of emotion, in willingness to disclose the injury to adults, and in how the symptoms are described. Younger children as compared to adolescents may be more likely to express their injury overtly (e.g., crying), thus making the injury more easily recognized by adults. Yet, this age-typical tearful behavior in the 5-year-old could be due to a number of possible causes (e.g., frustration or surprise at the collision) other than injury. The 15-year-old might be more inclined to decline the need for assistance and minimize the pain (e.g., stating, "I'm fine"), recognizing the likelihood of being pulled from play as a result. Yet, adolescents also possess greater capacity to articulate the injury and their symptoms. Understanding these developmental dynamics is important to a valid pediatric concussion evaluation.

Accurate evaluation of postconcussion symptoms requires developmentally appropriate assessment measures appropriate to the child's cognitive level, reading skill and vocabulary, and capacity to perceive their own symptoms accurately (Fritz et al. 1996). The reliability of symptom report in younger preadolescent children may be lower than for older reporters due to a variety of factors, including a concrete cognitive style, limited sense of time, lack of familiarity with symptom terminology, an affirmative response style to please the inquiring adult, greater difficulties judging "grades" of symptoms, and social–emotional maturity (De Los Reyes and Kazdin 2005; McCrea et al. 2004; Upton et al. 2008). Each of these factors must be taken into consideration when assessing symptoms in the younger child. Using developmentally appropriate language such as, "Does your head hurt?" instead of, "Do you have a headache?" is important, particularly for younger children. Similarly, more abstract terms such as "feeling foggy" (which appears on many symptom scales developed for adults) are not appropriate with younger children, nor are those symptoms involving complex vocabulary, perception of subtle internal states, sleep behaviors, and other items not likely to be monitored by younger children. Children also have greater difficulty linking events to abstract time terminology such as "yesterday," "last week," or even "*before* your injury." They are less adept at reporting accurately when an event occurred, thus it is important to make sure that presence of any symptoms is current, and not being recalled from a time point earlier in the injury or even before the injury! Similarly, the commonly used 7-point Likert scaling is abstract, and it is too complex a cognitive decision for younger children (Varni et al. 2007a; Fritz et al. 1996). A smaller number of choices (2 or 3 points) is more appropriate to their cognitive developmental level. Finally, the use of a visual analog scale (e.g., the Faces pain scale; Bieri et al. 1990) can be very helpful for assessment in younger children (Fritz et al. 1996), as it makes the numbered ratings more concrete. Given these developmental challenges in postconcussion assessment, it is important that parents serve as an additional and complementary source of information (Varni et al. 2007b).

12.2   Developmental Adaptation of a Pediatric Concussion Assessment Battery

In response to the dearth of work examining concussion outcomes in children less than age 13, the Centers for Disease Control and Prevention (CDC) funded the first author to construct developmentally appropriate standardized measures of neuropsychological function and postconcussion symptoms. Below we describe our development of the multi-informant set of symptom scales, the Post-Concussion Symptom Inventory (PCSI; Gioia et al. 2009a, b), and a computer administered neurocognitive test battery, Pediatric Immediate Post-Concussion Assessment and Cognitive Testing (Pediatric ImPACT; Gioia et al. 2011) for children ages 5–12 years (Gioia et al. 2009a; Gioia et al. 2011).

12.2.1   Pediatric ImPACT

Pediatric ImPACT is a developmental adaptation of the adolescent/adult ImPACT battery (Lovell et al. 2002). As mentioned in Chapter 10, the pediatric version of ImPACT consists of six subtests that tap cognitive functions related to concussion including episodic learning/memory and reaction time/processing speed. Each of the subtests was based on tasks included in the original ImPACT measure but with adaptations of task instructions, cognitive demands, stimuli, and format of the subtest appropriate to children age 5–12 years, including game-like story themes to make the tasks more engaging. Psychometric analyses of the battery ($n = 705$) highlight no systematic gender effects in performance but significant age-related differences in response speed ($r=-0.80$) and recognition memory ($r=0.43$) performance, emphasizing the importance of developmentally appropriate measures that take into account typical developmental variability.

12.2.2 Postconcussion Symptom Inventory

The PCSI was created to gather multiple informant input on symptom presentation. The 22-item symptom scale originally developed for adolescents and adults (Lovell et al. 2006) was adapted for parent and teacher report and for self-report by younger preadolescent children (Gioia et al. 2009a; Gioia et al. 2008b). Parent and teacher respondents are instructed to rate, using the 7-point Likert scaling, the degree to which 20 symptoms are observed in the home or school setting. The PCSI form asks for both a retrospective preinjury baseline report of symptoms and a postinjury report of symptoms observed over the past day. The PCSI is administered at each clinic visit to track symptom recovery. The Self-Report PCSI is administered to children in a similar manner as the parents (i.e., retrospective preinjury baseline report, current postinjury report). Developmentally specific PCSI forms are used appropriate to the age level of the child (age 5–7, 8–12, 13–18 years). The PCSI for the 5–7 age group was reduced to 13 symptoms, removing items with complex vocabulary, subtle internal states, sleep behaviors, and other items not likely monitored by younger children. The PCSI form for 8–12 year-olds includes most of the original 22 items with age appropriate adaptations, resulting in a 17-item inventory. Both of these rating scales were modified to a 3-point Likert scale asking whether the symptom is present "not at all," "a little," or "a lot." By contrast, the PCSI for the 13–18 age group children parallels the parent/teacher version in its wording and response format.

Research on child versus parent report of postconcussion symptoms indicates varying perspectives (Gioia et al. 2009b; Hajek et al. 2011). Using a sample of children and adolescents referred for assessment after concussive injury, parent-child agreement of symptom ratings differed by age (unpublished data). Concordance in our sample was highest in adolescents ($r=.68$), while children aged 8–12 exhibited less robust agreement but still significant associations (rs range from .25 to .45 for symptom clusters). In the youngest group (5–7 year-olds) little agreement was found between parent and child reports of physical and cognitive symptoms (rs < .3), with a marginal level of agreement for emotional symptoms. Further examination of the data indicated that, at times, parents reported the presence of symptoms that the younger children denied, perhaps because they were directly observable by an adult but not internally identifiable by a young child (e.g., fatigue). On the contrary, some symptoms were reported by children that their parents did not identify (e.g., sensitivity to light or noise). Therefore, particularly in younger children, multiple informants offer unique and valuable input into postconcussion symptom assessment.

An additional consideration is the possibility of gender differences in types of postconcussive symptoms. Preliminary support exists for gender differences in postconcussion symptoms (Frommer et al. 2011), substantiating the need for further research in this area. In the sample described above, we found that girls generally experience higher levels of concussion symptoms than boys, and that this finding is consistent across both parent and self-ratings. Parent ratings ($n = 548$) were higher for injured girls than boys across symptom clusters assessing emotional, cognitive, fatigue, and somatic/physical symptoms; these differences were most pronounced in adolescents. On self-reports ($n = 691$), there was a similar interaction of age and gender, such that female adolescents reported a higher level of symptoms (particularly for somatic and cognitive symptom clusters) than their male counterparts, with symptom ratings more similar between younger boys and girls. The presence of more pronounced gender differences with age needs further investigation, and raises questions of whether hormones, personality styles, neurobiological effects, or mechanics of injury are at play. Notably, there were few differences in injury characteristics (e.g., presence of LOC and amnesias) between males and females, so acute injury factors cannot explain the differences found. Moreover, gender differences were not identified in a separate sample of noninjured children and adolescents (both parent and self-ratings), underscoring the possibility that postconcussion gender differences are related to girls' unique response to the injury.

12.3   Evaluation of Concussion Across the Injury Timeline

As recovery from concussion is a dynamic process, evaluation and management require an understanding of the changing manifestations along the recovery continuum. The elapsed time since injury is one of the most important considerations as this influences the goals and methods of the evaluation. Recovery from concussion is a dynamic process that has been described in three stages (Kirkwood et al. 2008): acute (first 3 days), postacute (3 days – 3 months), and long-term (greater than 3 months) for those with persisting symptoms. Since symptoms typically change rapidly after injury, a flexible model of evaluation and monitoring is necessary, from the immediate postinjury stage to final recovery. Table 12.1 highlights the associated personnel, service goals, clinical tools, and indications for referral at the acute and postacute stages of recovery. For example, the goals of evaluation and management in the acute stage are recognizing the injury, stabilizing the child, and providing basic postinjury guidance to parents, teachers, and the student (Gioia et al. 2008a). During the postacute stage, the goals shift to a more in-depth assessment of symptom and neurocognitive manifestations in the service of planning for active treatment (Kirkwood et al. 2008). Note that evaluation at this stage does not typically require a comprehensive neuropsychological assessment. Although the majority of concussions recover within 3 months (McCrea 2008), persisting symptoms beyond this time indicate the need for a more comprehensive evaluation of neurologic, neuropsychological, and social–emotional functions to identify the factors

Table 12.1 Concussion management service with associated personnel, goals, clinical tools, and referral indications

Service	Personnel	Service goals		Clinical tools		Indications for referral/additional evaluation
		Evaluation	Management	Evaluation	Management	
Acute stage						
Early Recognition/Identification Fieldside Roadside Home	Nonmedical *Parent Coach Peer/Sibling*	First Aid: Recognize/Suspect	*Respond/Protect:* When in Doubt, Sit Them Out *Refer* for medical evaluation	CDC Signs and Symptoms materials (Clipboard, Fact Sheet, Pocket Card, Phone App)	ACE Home/School Instructions	If any reasonable suspicion of blow to head with signs or symptoms
School Community	Medical *School Nurse Athletic Trainer EMT Physician*	Acute Evaluation of signs and symptoms, mental status; diagnosis	Early symptom management; reduce stimulation; contact family, primary care or emergency care	ACE/CDC SAC BESS/balance SCAT2	ACE Home/School Instructions	Reasonable suspicion or confirmation of the diagnosis
Emergency Medical Care	Triage Nurse PNP ED physician	Diagnosis, stabilization	Early symptom management; educate; reduce stimulation; refer for follow-up with primary care	ACE-ED	ACE-ED Home/School Instructions	Confirmation of the diagnosis
Postacute stage						
Concussion Generalist	Triage Nurse PNP Physician Certified Athletic Trainer Other Trained Healthcare Provider	Diagnosis, assess risk factors for prolonged recovery, tracking of recovery	Ongoing symptom management; educate; reduced activity in home and school; guidance for school and sports	ACE SCAT2 SAC/BESS	ACE Home/School Instructions; ACE Care Plan	Persistent symptoms (greater than 5–7 days) with little improvement; school programming, athletic RTP
Concussion Specialist	Physician Neuropsychologist Certified Athletic Trainer	Confirm concussion diagnosis and establish comorbid diagnoses, assess risk factors/comorbidities, including activity level, response to exertion	Active symptom management; educate; engage in increasing managed activity; establish readiness for Return to Play/Return to Risk ADL's	ACE SAC/SCAT2 Neuropsychological testing Balance testing (MRI, EEG, etc.)	ACE Care Plan; Individualized treatment letters	Atypical persisting neurological, neuropsychological or psychiatric symptoms.

associated with poor recovery progress. Thus, clarifying goals for the concussion evaluation at each recovery stage helps frame an approach and appropriate methods (Kirkwood et al. 2008; Turkstra et al. 2005).

We advocate a stage-specific approach using developmentally sensitive and validated tools to facilitate assessment and management of concussion in children, stressing the unique goals of the pediatric postinjury recovery process in returning to home life, school, and sports/recreation activities. Previous chapters in this book (Chapters 5 and 6) have addressed in greater detail the evaluation and management at the acute stage, including field side identification, emergency medical care, and primary care service. The acute stages are, therefore, briefly reviewed with respect to the unique features presented by the developing child before turning greater attention to the postacute stage.

12.3.1   Acute Stage: Early Recognition/Identification

Early recognition and identification of a pediatric concussion is THE critical first step towards facilitating a speedy recovery and reducing the chance of an adverse outcome. The challenge lies in recognizing two primary events (1) a blow to the head or body that produces rapid acceleration/deceleration of the head; and (2) emergence of temporally associated and relevant signs or symptoms.

12.3.1.1   Service Goals

For the nonmedical personnel, the goal at this stage is to *recognize* the concussion or, at the very least, suspect that it has occurred, and to *respond* with an appropriate action plan. The goal for nonmedical personnel is *not* to diagnose a concussion but, instead, to observe that the blow to the child's head resulted in a change in their functioning. The management goal at this point is to remove the child from any further danger (i.e., sitting them out of the sports practice or game) and seek further medical evaluation to determine whether a concussion has occurred.

The first-responder medical personnel would be capable of a more active clinical examination. The goal of the evaluation would be to assess the acute signs and symptoms, and mental status as well as to conduct a neurological evaluation, rendering a diagnosis in some cases. Initial management recommendations (in addition to removing the child from additional danger) might include acute symptom management, reduced stimulation, and careful observation for the purpose of triaging to a more intensive medical setting if necessary and contacting the family, emergency care, or primary care medical providers.

12.3.1.2 Personnel

The personnel present at this stage are often times not trained professionals but instead are bystanders at the sporting or recreational event or happen to be at the scene (school, home, field side, roadside, community) where the injury takes place. This might be a parent, coach, teammate, sibling, or friend. Preparation of these persons with key first aid knowledge of the injury is, therefore, essential to early recognition.

In certain situations, there may be a medical professional on the scene who can conduct an early assessment. These first responders might be an athletic trainer, school nurse, emergency medical technician, or a sideline physician.

12.3.1.3 Clinical Tools

An increasing library of materials is being developed to educate parents, coaches, athletes, teachers, and others to recognize and respond to a suspected concussion. The "Heads Up" toolkits produced by the Centers for Disease Control and Prevention (CDC) are a rich source of information to guide recognition by the nonclinician. Specifically, the Signs and Symptoms chart on clipboard stickers, pocket cards, and Parent/Coach Fact Sheets are very useful aids. Initial management instructions can be found on the ACE Home/ School Instructions sheet, adapted from the published ACE Care Plan (CDC 2007).

The medical provider also has several tools at their disposal for evaluation of a possible concussion including the CDC toolkit's Acute Concussion Evaluation (ACE), the Sport Concussion Assessment Tool, 2nd Ed (SCAT2), or the Sideline Assessment of Concussion (SAC), as well as balance assessment (Guskiewicz et al. 2001).

One challenge to early recognition is determining whether there is a "difference" from the child's typical or baseline functional state, i.e., reliably detecting change from "usual" functioning. Depending on the child's age and preinjury functioning, detecting such change may be difficult. For example, it may be difficult to detect a change in attentional functioning in a child with preinjury attention deficits or in a very young child. Detecting a change in irritability or sadness in an individual with preinjury anxiety or depression may also be a challenge. Direct questioning of the patient or caretaker about their observations of any changes from the child's usual state of functioning can be particularly useful. A second challenge may be to determine whether an observed change is related to the force taken by the brain rather than to a nonconcussion related event (e.g., dehydration, neck injury). Because of these complexities, the untrained layperson should always follow the first aid safety rule "When in doubt, sit them out."

12.3.1.4 Indications for Referral/Additional Evaluation

Any reasonable evidence of a blow to the head or body resulting in concussion signs or symptoms should be referred for further medical evaluation. The evaluation tools provide the patient and family with guidance regarding cardinal signs and symptoms that would prompt immediate emergency medical evaluation.

12.3.2 Acute Stage: Emergency Medical Care

As with most injuries, the presentation of concussion can be quite obvious or quite subtle, and the recovery process varies widely in length of time. As discussed in Chapter 6, the emergency department (ED) plays a specific role in medical care serving as the frontline for the acutely injured. ED clinicians are charged with the task of making accurate and timely diagnoses, differentiating a concussion from a more severe medical emergency (e.g., epidural or subdural hematoma, neck injury), and providing appropriate initial management including following up with the primary care system to provide for continuity of care.

The ED differs from primary medical care settings with respect to evaluation and management of concussion. Differences exist with respect to service goals, functions, and processes. The two settings differ in the reasons for referral, based often on the acuity and level of risk presented by the initial signs and symptoms. Referral to the ED is most appropriate when there is a question of significant trauma with life-threatening potential, presentation with multiple trauma (e.g., suspected orthopedic or spinal injuries) or significant neurological signs (loss of consciousness, significant or persistent confusion/amnesia, focal neurologic signs, persistent vomiting). By contrast, referral to the primary care physician (PCP) is more typical with a lower-risk injury without significant trauma or risk of catastrophic outcome, such as when the patient presents nonacutely with more typical postconcussion signs (headache, dizziness).

12.3.2.1 Service Goals

The service goals of the ED are to establish an initial diagnosis, stabilize the child's medical condition, reduce mortality and morbidity, and provide short-term management with guidance for follow-up with the PCP. In doing so, key symptoms and signs are evaluated to rule out more significant neuropathology. Management is largely organized around these major symptoms, as well as guiding the patient/family to be able to identify the "danger signs" associated with possible neurological deterioration that would prompt the need for return to the ED. Examination, diagnosis, and management in the ED typically involves a brief examination of an unknown patient by gathering limited basic medical and injury history to assist the primary clinical goal of diagnosis and stabilization. The ED will not typically schedule their own clinical follow-up but instead will communicate their evaluation, diagnosis, and early management plan to the primary care medical providers. With respect to management from the ED, prescribing a predetermined period of nonparticipation from sports (e.g., "You may return to sports after 7 days.") at this acute phase postinjury is *not* appropriate as it is difficult to predict individual recovery at this time. Return to sports or any high risk activity can be dangerous if premature. Rather, proscribing any return to sports or high risk activity until further evaluation by the primary care system is appropriate.

12.3.2.2 Personnel

To meet the significant service demands of the emergency department setting, the personnel are trained to evaluate and treat a wide range of medical conditions. The triage nurse, emergency medicine physician, and nurse practitioner typically compose the personnel in the ED.

12.3.2.3 Clinical Tools

The ACE- Emergency Department (ACE-ED) was adapted from the original ACE (Gioia et al. 2008a) to assist in the identification and diagnosis of concussion. It provides a standardized assessment format to assist in defining the injury and associated characteristics within the broader understanding of the patient's immediate history and presentation to facilitate an appropriate diagnosis. The instrument is administered as a clinical interview of the patient directly and/or of a knowledgeable caretaker as part of a clinical exam. The ACE-ED is organized according to key areas of inquiry, including (1) specific characteristics of the injury including details of the direct or indirect blow to the head, retrograde and anterograde amnesia and loss of consciousness; (2) fourteen symptoms and four signs associated with concussion, referred to as the ACE Symptom Checklist; and (3) three key risk factors that might modify the concussion recovery (e.g., history of previous concussion and migraine headaches).

The ACE Home/School Instructions were developed to guide the process of early postconcussion management of daily life, adjusting school demands, work demands, and return-to-sports and recreation as needed. Avoidance of activities that could lead to a second injury remains paramount, but the fundamental concepts driving treatment recommendations are maximizing rest and minimizing overexertion of brain activity during recovery. Excessive physical and/or mental activity frequently can result in an increase in symptoms (i.e., exertional effects) and can be counterproductive to recovery. Student-athletes and persons with demanding school and/or work responsibilities can experience significant cognitive exertional effects with adverse effects on academic and/or work function, and may have prolonged recovery if not appropriately managed. With these essentials in mind, the ACE Home/School Instructions offer specific recommendations regarding return to school, work, sports and return to home life/social activities.

Table 12.2 Determinants of concussion generalist and specialist services

		Recovery	
		Typical/ Progressive	Atypical/Nonprogressive
Reinjury risk	Low	Concussion generalist	Concussion specialist
	High	Generalist (with Specialist input for return)	Specialist

12.3.2.4   Indications for Referral/Additional Evaluation

Following diagnosis and initial stabilization of the child, the next important step of the Emergency Medical Care system is to refer the patient and family to the primary care medical system for follow-up care.

12.3.3   Postacute Stage

Evaluation and management of concussions at the postacute stage can be performed competently by a variety of disciplines with appropriate, injury-specific, training including nurses, physicians, athletic trainers, psychologists, and neuropsychologists (see Chapters 8 and 9 for further discussion of evaluation at the postacute stage). Several factors related to the injury presentation must, however, be considered in determining the type and level of evaluation. Below, we differentiate between "concussion generalist" and "concussion specialist" evaluation and management, which require different levels of training and expertise. Table 12.2 presents this distinction as determined by the (1) type of recovery (typical/progressive versus atypical/nonprogressive), and (2) risk of reinjury (high versus low) in returning to everyday activities. Recovery in most concussions is progressive with regular improvement in symptoms over time. Although it is difficult to specify a "typical" timeframe for recovery, in the uncomplicated pattern the child or adolescent makes steady progress over time toward baseline levels of functioning with complete resolution of symptoms. By contrast, the atypical/nonprogressive recovery pattern can be defined in several ways: an irregular time frame that either results in a prolonged period of recovery, a lack of steady progress, or the presence of atypical or idiosyncratic symptoms (e.g., speech dysfluency, persistent visual problems, reports of total loss of preinjury memory).

Risk of reinjury is defined as the likelihood that the child or adolescent would be reinjured upon return to normal activity. Although there is arguably risk in any activity, children that play contact or collision sports or engage regularly in certain dangerous behaviors (e.g., impulsive or aggressive behavior) would be considered at high risk for reinjury, necessitating greater certainty that they are fully recovered. For example, a football or soccer player is returning to a higher risk activity than a swimmer and, therefore, the decision to return demands greater certainty of full recovery.

12.3.3.1 Concussion Generalist Service

Many children and adolescents with concussions can be evaluated by the "concussion generalist." From a public health perspective, given the increasing recognition of suspected concussions, there is a need to increase the number of trained professionals conducting concussion generalist services. A variety of medical and sports organizations as well as the Centers for Disease Control and Prevention (CDC) are currently striving towards improving the general education and skills of pediatric practitioners to do so. When a child is injured, most parents call their primary care physician (PCP) for answers to questions about their child's medical condition. In some regions, other medical professionals may be available to provide early postacute follow-up including sports medicine physicians, neuropsychologists, or certified athletic trainers. The concussion generalist is typically a clinician who is available to conduct the initial evaluation early after the injury. In most cases, the PCP will be the first point of contact and may choose to perform the concussion evaluation immediately, or a triage examination might determine that a referral to the emergency medical system in appropriate. Examination of the child by the PCP is typically appropriate for lower-risk, uncomplicated injuries without significant trauma or risk of catastrophic outcome, where the patient presents nonacutely with common postinjury symptoms (headache, dizziness, etc.).

Service Goals

The primary service goal of the concussion generalist's evaluation is to establish or confirm the diagnosis if already rendered on the sideline or in the ED. The primary care setting affords relatively more time than in the ED to comprehensively assess concussion signs and symptoms. The concussion evaluation in this setting, therefore, allows for a more thorough clinical evaluation with the goal of ongoing monitoring and management until symptom resolution and recovery. Oftentimes, the PCP has the benefit of knowing the patient's medical history, which can be integrated with the diagnosis and management plan. The primary care office, in general, has a greater capacity for regular clinical follow-up and injury management. The focus of management is to assure that premature return to activities that place the child at risk does not occur, to monitor and manage symptoms, to educate the patient and family with regard to the injury and its management, and to monitor response to treatment recommendations. Guidance should be provided with respect to home, school, and sports/recreation activities.

Personnel

With respect to professional skill level, the concussion generalist service requires general knowledge and experience in concussion evaluation and management and availability to a fundamental set of assessment tools (symptom-based) and treatment methods. Any healthcare provider with the appropriate training, knowledge and skills to provide early postacute evaluation and ongoing management of concussion may serve in the role of concussion generalist. Examples of such disciplines might include the PCP, nurse practitioner, and primary care sports medicine physician; although, depending on the resources available in various geographic regions, other healthcare providers may provide this service as well.

Clinical Tools

The concussion generalist has several tools at their disposal for evaluation of a possible concussion. The CDC physician's toolkit includes the Acute Concussion Evaluation (ACE; Gioia et al. 2008a), a systematic protocol for assessing concussion. The ACE is organized according to key areas of inquiry, including (1) specific characteristics of the injury including details of the direct or indirect blow to the head, retrograde and anterograde amnesia and loss of consciousness; (2) a full array of 22 symptoms and five signs associated with concussion, referred to as the ACE Symptom Checklist; and (3) premorbid risk factors that might predict a prolonged recovery. The presence of these risk factors would prompt the clinician to expect a lengthier recovery period and to counsel the patient about this possibility, or to refer onto a concussion specialist with the anticipation that the injury recovery may be complicated. The ACE also serves as a tool for monitoring the array of symptoms over time through repeated assessments. Serial assessment can document the progress of recovery or, with little or no progress, prompt referral to a specialist (e.g., neuropsychologist for neuropsychological assessment, neurologist for more in-depth examination of neurologic function) for further in depth evaluation. In addition to the ACE, tools developed for sport-related concussion include the Sport Concussion Assessment Tool, 2nd Ed (SCAT2), or the Sideline Assessment of Concussion (SAC), and balance assessment (Halstead and Walter 2010). Some concussion generalists may have access to neuropsychological assessment or consultation as part of the evaluation process, although many do not.

Management tools include the ACE Home/School Instructions for the early days of recovery, and the ACE Care Plan (CDC 2007) that educates and guides recovery in the home, school, and recreation/sports settings. The ACE Care Plan provides specific academic accommodations and return to play guidelines that can be individualized based on a particular child's needs during recovery.

Indications for Referral/Additional Evaluation

Referral to a concussion specialist is indicated when the recovery pattern is more complicated, e.g., atypical symptom presentation, complications/exacerbation of premorbid headaches or emotional difficulties, symptoms persist without noticeable change over 1 week, issues related to detailed school recommendations are raised, or there is a return to high risk activities (e.g., contact sport) where the protocol exists that includes neuropsychological testing as a component in the Return to Play (RTP) decision.

12.3.3.2 Concussion Specialist Service

As noted above, when the child's recovery pattern becomes more complex in terms of the length of time or the presence of atypical factors, the concussion specialist service is necessary.

Service Goals

The primary goals of the concussion specialist's evaluation are to confirm the diagnosis, to understand the reasons for an atypical recovery pattern including assessment of risk factors and comorbid diagnoses, as well as to define the types of management that have taken place to date (activity level, response to exertion). The goals of concussion management are to develop an active treatment plan based on evaluation data, to educate the patient and family regarding the specific factors contributing to the delayed recovery, to guide implementation of management and treatment plans, and to monitor their success.

Personnel

The concussion specialist is differentiated from the generalist in several ways. The concussion specialist service necessitates more in-depth training, knowledge, and experience with brain injury across the spectrum of severity; subspecialty training in a brain injury-related field (e.g., physiatry, neurology, neuropsychology, neurosurgery, sports medicine); training in the differential diagnosis of competing disorders (e.g., ADHD, depression, seizures); and the availability of an advanced set of assessment tools (e.g., neuropsychological testing, neuroimaging, EEG) and treatments. Given the complexity of the brain and its injury, no single medical discipline possesses in-depth knowledge and skill in evaluating and treating all its manifestations, requiring a respectful and active collaboration of complementary professional skill sets.

Clinical Tools

While the concussion specialist has available to them the same clinical tools as the generalist (e.g., ACE, SAC/SCAT2), they also have access to additional tools to conduct the more in-depth assessments required to understand the complexity of an irregular recovery pattern. These tools include such methods as neuropsychological testing, neuroimaging, neurological assessment, postural stability/balance testing, and psychiatric evaluation.

Indications for Referral/Additional Evaluation

The concussion specialist may also consider additional referrals when other factors are discovered beyond their expertise. For example, if a particular pattern of visual disturbance is identified by the neurologist or neuropsychologist, referral to a neuroophthalmologist might be indicated. Common persisting issues requiring further referral can include disordered sleep, chronic persisting headaches, mood or anxiety problems, and significant cognitive dysfunction such as inattention or poor memory.

The concussion specialist's clinical evaluation assists in clarifying the diagnosis of concussion as well as possible comorbid diagnoses by specifying and differentiating the injury's symptom manifestation from noninjury factors, including preexisting developmental, cognitive, emotional, and physical impairments. At this level of care, specialized knowledge of all levels of brain injury severity and competing comorbid conditions is necessary. As such, the individual conducting the specialist evaluation has additional diagnostic expertise in areas of sensory/motor, balance, vestibular and other neurologic dysfunction (i.e., neurologist, neurosurgeon), neurocognitive/neurobehavioral function such as attentional/learning deficits or mood disorders (i.e., neuropsychologist) to understand these issues in the context of the concussive injury. The concussion specialist evaluation also specifies the breadth and severity of the postconcussion symptom profile. The evaluation explores the complexity of possible contributing factors, including the role of family, school, or other environmental factors that can facilitate or impede recovery (e.g., excessive cognitive exertion in school). To explore these issues, the concussion specialist has advanced assessment tools at their disposal such as neuropsychological testing or neuroimaging. The specialist also has advanced knowledge about treatment related to these contributory factors (management of cognitive activity).

12.4   Fundamental Components of the Concussion Evaluation

Evaluation of a pediatric concussion, at the generalist or specialist level, involves the assessment of six fundamental components: (1) definition of the injury's characteristics, (2) history of premorbid and postinjury risk factors, (3) current neurocognitive functioning, (4) detailed assessment of postconcussion symptoms, (5) balance assessment, and (6) examination of social–emotional functioning. The evaluation should also assess family functioning as well as the effects of the injury on school performance and social/recreational activity (Camiolo Reddy et al. 2008). The evaluation process involves serial assessment and monitoring of postconcussion symptom recovery with active guidance of gradual return to school and play/sports.

12.4.1   Injury Definition and Characteristics

Defining the acute injury characteristics is important to frame the severity and possible risks of the injury, including a description of the injury and the types of forces involved, mechanism of injury, location (e.g., frontal or temporal) of the blow, evidence of alteration of conscious and/or confusion, presence of retrograde and anterograde amnesia, seizure activity, early signs and symptoms, and radiologic findings. Postinjury signs such as retrograde amnesia or confusion can be important as they have been shown to be predictive of later neurocognitive dysfunction and protracted symptom resolution (Lovell et al. 2003).

12.4.2   Preinjury History

It is critical to obtain a good clinical history of preinjury functioning from the patient, family, and when possible teachers accompanied by any available documentation in the medical and school records. A thorough developmental history, medical/neurological history (including personal/ family history of chronic headaches), school history, and psychiatric history (including sleep disorders, anxiety, depression) provides essential information about the child's preinjury functioning, risk factors such as premorbid learning, attentional, psychiatric, or behavioral disorders, familial risks for the same, and family environment. In addition, the clinician should gather a detailed history of previous concussions/brain injuries including age at injury, injury characteristics, and length of symptoms and neurocognitive dysfunction.

12.4.3   Postconcussion Symptoms

A thorough assessment of postconcussion symptoms is an essential component of the evaluation. The four symptom types – physical, cognitive, emotional, and sleep-related – should be fully explored in terms of their presence, severity, and change over time. It is most useful to track symptoms from the onset of injury to the time of the evaluation to understand the rate of recovery and assess the degree and type of impact that the injury is having on the child's life. This assessment should include collecting structured symptom ratings from the parents and the injured child (Gioia et al. 2009b).

12.4.4   Neurocognitive Functions

Neurocognitive testing provides an objective, quantifiable set of data that is sensitive in detecting the often subtle effects (e.g., reaction time) of a concussion. Specific neurocognitive domains have demonstrated sensitivity to the effects of concussion – attention/concentration, working memory, speed of processing, and learning/ memory, and the executive functions (Catroppa et al. 2007; Babikian and Asarnow 2009; Schatz et al. 2006). Focused, targeted neuropsychological testing of key neurocognitive domains can be an important component in the postacute stage of pediatric concussion (Kirkwood et al. 2008), particularly when return to play (i.e., high risk return) decisions are pending. Additionally, the student's profile of cognitive performance obtained from the neuropsychological assessment can also be useful to guiding the management of school learning.

Two basic approaches to postacute neuropsychological testing are common: paper and pencil and computerized measures, each method having its strengths and limitations. Paper and pencil-based tests have demonstrated appropriate sensitivity to the effects of concussion (McCrea et al. 2005; Echemendia and Julian 2001). They pose psychometric limitations, however, making them less ideal for serial assessment in that many of these tests lack equivalent alternative forms, are susceptible to interrater biases, and show significant practice effects (Collie et al. 2001). They may also be less able to detect the subtle changes in reaction time and processing speed (Maroon et al. 2000).

Computer-administered tests (Collie and Maruff 2003; Lovell 2008) allow for alternate randomized forms and serial tracking of recovery with limited or known practice effects. They can be parameterized to increase sensitivity to mild cognitive dysfunction, incorporating precise reaction time to the hundredth of a second (McCrory et al. 2005). Computer-based measures, however, have the disadvantage of constrained response options – e.g., allowing only recognition memory responses versus free recall format. Currently, four computer-based management approaches have been developed to assist concussion management and return to play issues after concussion, including ImPACT (Immediate Post-Concussion Assessment and Cognitive Testing), CogState (CogSport), Headminders, and ANAM (Automated Neurocognitive Assessment Metrics). Each of these test batteries has examined important aspects of reliability and validity in their approach to measuring concussive injury. Specific computerized test batteries have published additional data examining sensitivity/specificity of their test battery and the "added value" of their assessment tool when compared with the assessment of symptoms in isolation (Schatz et al. 2006; van Kampen et al. 2006; Fazio et al. 2007).

Neuropsychological testing is not always available in the concussion evaluation, necessitating an alternative approach to the assessment of cognitive functioning. Interviewing the child and parent, reviewing grades/school performance, talking to teachers or other care providers all are valuable clinical means of assessing any deviation in the child's cognitive functioning at home and school. As this assessment method is less precise than testing, a more conservative approach to concussion recovery and return-to-activity must be taken.

12.4.5 Balance/Postural Stability

Postural stability has been demonstrated to be an objective element in the evaluation of athletes with acute concussion (Guskiewicz et al. 1996). Concussion can disrupt the various sensory systems, including the visual, somatosensory, and vestibular systems. Concussed collegiate athletes exhibited an increase in postural sway with decreases in postural stability persisting for up to 3 days following injury.

Postural stability assessment, through the use of force plate technology or a clinical balance test such as the Balance Error Scoring System (BESS; Riemann et al. 1999; Riemann and Guskiewicz 2000), may be useful in identifying neurologic impairment in student-athletes (see further discussion of the BESS in Chap. 5). Several postural-stability tests have been used to assess balance following concussion, including basic tests of balance and coordination such as the Romberg and stork stand. The BESS was developed as a clinical measure to assess impaired balance using three stance positions on a firm and a foam surface with the eyes closed. The BESS has established appropriate test-retest reliability and evidence of validity when compared with laboratory forceplate measures (Guskiewicz et al. 2001; Riemann et al. 1999) in injured versus control groups. Little systematic research on postural stability has been conducted, however, in the preadolescent child (Gagnon et al. 2004).

12.4.6 Social–Emotional Functioning

Social, emotional, and behavioral functioning can be impaired following concussion (Mainwaring et al. 2004), including increased irritability, sadness, or over-emotionality. Basic symptom rating scales can be used to screen for these issues. In addition, clinical interview of everyday functioning (i.e., depression, anxiety, somatic concerns, atypical behaviors, etc.) from parents, teachers, and the child can be useful. Several standardized behavior rating scales such as the Child Behavior Checklist can be useful to evaluate pre- and postinjury behavioral, social, and emotional functioning, capturing broadband problems (Satz et al. 1997).

12.4.7 Modifying Factors

The evaluation must also explore factors that have the potential of modifying recovery outcomes. In general, severity of the injury within the mild TBI category has been shown to be associated with outcome (Hessen et al. 2006) with more severe injury characteristics (e.g., "complicated" mild TBI) resulting in higher risk for long-term neuropsychological dysfunction (Fay et al. 2009; Taylor et al. 2010). Age at injury likely plays a role in time to recovery (Babikian and Asarnow 2009; McKinlay et al. 2002) as high school athletes may require longer time to recover than collegiate and professional athletes (Field et al. 2003; Moser et al. 2005; Pellman et al. 2006) and younger children may recover more slowly than older children (McKinlay et al. 2002). Collins and colleagues (2006) report at least 25% of high school football players taking up to 4 weeks to reach recovery criteria, well beyond what is reported for older athletes. Additional factors reported as possible modifiers of recovery outcome include a premorbid history of learning and behavioral problems (Collins et al. 1999; Light et al. 1998; Massagli et al. 2004; Ponsford et al. 1999), history of chronic headaches (Mihalik et al. 2005), and history of previous concussions (Collins et al. 2002; Ponsford et al. 1999; Swaine et al. 2007;

Iverson et al. 2006). The family expectations and functioning (Anderson et al. 2001; Hawley et al. 2003) and type of postinjury activity management (Majerske et al. 2008; Comper et al. 2005; Ponsford et al. 2001) have also been associated with recovery outcomes. The "cognitive reserve" model may help to explain why the child with these premorbid disorders is at higher risk for a prolonged recovery. The basic concept is that the presence of these premorbid factors results in fewer degrees of freedom to support a faster recovery. Fay et al. (2010) posited that postconcussive symptom presentation in children may be associated with cognitive reserve capacity. They found children of lower cognitive ability with complicated mild TBI were more prone to cognitive symptoms across time and to high levels of postconcussion symptoms in the acute period (Fay et al. 2010).

12.4.8   Determining Deviation from Baseline

A challenge in the clinical evaluation of concussion is to distinguish change from preinjury functioning. As noted previously, normal developmental change must be taken into account. One must determine that the child's symptoms and neuropsychological functioning are different from their "normal" baseline. In some cases, general baseline data may be available from prior evaluations if the child was evaluated for educational purposes. Baseline data are also increasingly available from preseason assessments for the students involved in sports. The baseline assessment model posits that capturing neurocognitive functioning preinjury serves as a specific benchmark against which postinjury functioning can be compared using reliable change metrics to identify the likelihood of clinically significant differences in performance and symptoms. In most cases, though, no baseline test data is available, requiring other strategies for estimation of preinjury functioning. One strategy for estimating return to baseline functioning involves serial tracking of cognitive performance and symptom reports to establish improvements in functioning, or a recovery curve. Additionally, one can conduct a thorough assessment of the child's developmental status to determine a general expectation of their level of functioning and any likely functional variability (such as lowered verbal skills with learning disabilities or inattention with ADHD). In addition, one can assess any observed changes from typical everyday functioning in home and school settings via parent, teacher, and self-report.

12.5   Case Illustration

Keira is an otherwise healthy 9-year-old girl in the fourth grade with no reported developmental, familial, or medical risk factors. She presented for a concussion specialist evaluation 3 weeks after sustaining her first concussion, striking the left temporal region of her head on a teammate's knee during a soccer game. There was no loss of consciousness but she was immediately removed from the game where her coach and parents observed her on the sidelines, referencing the signs and symptoms on the CDC clipboard that the team carries to each game and practice. She was confused in describing the events of the game and her injury, was speaking more slowly than usual, complained of a headache, and reported feeling nauseated. She was taken to the local Emergency Department (ED), where she received an acute evaluation using the Acute Concussion Evaluation-Emergency Department version (ACE-ED). Following observation in the ED, a CT scan of the brain was not deemed necessary. The collection of signs and symptoms associated with the blow to the head resulted in the diagnosis of a concussion, and was later useful for tracking her injury recovery. Keira and her family were referred to their pediatrician for follow-up care.

The pediatrician conducted a concussion generalist evaluation using the Acute Concussion Evaluation (ACE), assessing the four categories of symptoms. A host of somatic (headache, fatigue, sensitivity to light and sound), cognitive (troubles concentrating, feeling slowed down), and emotional (irritability) symptoms were identified. Her parents reported these symptoms to be out of character for Keira. Recommendations were made for reduced physical and cognitive activity, including accommodations at school, using the ACE Care Plan. Periodic monitoring of these symptoms by the pediatrician over a 2 week period revealed persisting headaches, fatigue and concentration difficulties, prompting a referral for a specialist evaluation. In the meantime, Keira had started school ten days postinjury. Her teacher observed that Keira often required redirection for inattention, fatigued easily, complained of headaches and the lights bothering her. No initial academic concerns were identified in reading, writing, or math skills although school had just restarted. The goals for the concussion specialist evaluation were to identify the range and severity of symptoms and neurocognitive dysfunction, the types and level of activities that worsened her symptoms, establish a plan to manage those symptoms and the associated activities, and guide return-to-school and physical activity.

The specialist evaluation included a thorough definition of the events of the injury, current postconcussion symptoms and behaviors, and a review of preinjury history including prior school performance. Keira's parents provided the background history and completed the PCSI for current symptoms as well as a retrospective report of preinjury symptoms. Keira completed PCSI appropriate for 9 year olds, assisted by the clinic staff. She completed a battery of paper-and-pencil and computerized neuropsychological tests to assess her attention, memory and processing speed. Change in symptom level associated with her cognitive exertion in clinic was directly assessed before and after testing using a visual analog scale to rate headache, fatigue, concentration, and irritability symptoms.

The neuropsychological assessment was remarkable for variable attention and slowed speed of processing with generally appropriate learning and memory performance when compared with her age mates. There was no preinjury baseline testing for direct comparison but her below average processing speed scores and her observed attentional difficulties in the context of a normally developing girl suggested impairment. In addition, her headache, fatigue and concentration symptoms worsened following the hour of cognitive testing, reflecting a sensitivity to cognitive exertion.

In assessing her symptoms, Keira reported an increased level relative to preinjury baseline as did her parents for concentration, headache, fatigue, irritability, and slowed thinking. Interview revealed that her sleep schedule was appropriate, although she would awaken in the morning still feeling tired. At school, she was not receiving any scheduled rest breaks and was consistently fatiguing by mid-morning with an increase in her headaches and concentration difficulties. She was eating lunch in the noisy cafeteria, which was bothering her. When she came home, she would engage in her normal routine of doing her homework right away even though she was significantly fatigued. Homework was, therefore, taking a significantly longer period of time. She attended her late afternoon 90 min soccer practices to observe although she did not play. On the weekends, assessment of her social and recreational activity schedule had revealed that although Keira's family initially reduced the overall schedule, she had increased it significantly with little opportunity for rest. The specialist evaluation identified Keira's specific symptom profile, the neurocognitive dysfunction as well as triggers for symptom exacerbation.

A number of opportunities were identified in the specialist evaluation for active management of Keira's recovery to balance her cognitive, physical and social activity with appropriate recovery. It was clear that she was overexerting throughout the school day and at home with little opportunity to rest formally in either setting, and no active monitoring of symptom exacerbation to guide her rest breaks. Keira and her family were educated about the concussion and the direct effects of the excessive activity on the brain's underlying neurometabolism. The concepts of physical and cognitive exertion were defined and operationalized, and the use of the exertional rating scale during testing was demonstrated for use at home and school. Symptom "safe" (i.e., below Keira's symptom threshold) levels of activity and an appropriate schedule of rest breaks at home and school were defined and articulated in the ACE Care Plan. Two subsequent clinic visits over the next three weeks reviewed Keira's progress, adjusted her accommodations allowing increasing levels of noncontact activity in school and at home. When fully asymptomatic at her last visit, the gradual return to play protocol was initiated under the supervision of a local sports rehabilitation program, and Keira returned to soccer after successfully performing the 1-week progressive program.

12.6 Key Points

Evaluation and management of concussion in the child and adolescent require a developmentally appropriate clinical model, emphasizing key factors relevant to the injury manifestation and needs of the child.

Key considerations in pediatric concussion evaluation and management include a core understanding of: normal development and application to the injured child, the child's capacity to fully engage in the evaluation and treatment, the central involvement of others such as parents, developmentally appropriate assessment measures, and the life demands of the child at home and school to develop an age-appropriate management plan.

A developmentally adapted standardized pediatric concussion assessment battery for children is described, including a new neurocognitive measure and PCSI completed by the child and parent.

The clinical model of pediatric concussion incorporates the full injury timeline from the acute through the postacute stages including key personnel, service goals, and available clinical tools.

Various disciplines contribute to the evaluation and management of concussion. The concept of the concussion generalist and specialist service is introduced with suggested requisite training, skills, and knowledge to evaluate and manage the full range of complexity of pediatric concussion. No single discipline possesses the entire knowledge and skill set to examine all types and complexities of concussions, requiring respectful collaboration between professionals.

References

Anderson, V., Catroppa, C., Morse, S., et al. (2001). Outcome from mild head injury in young children: a prospective study. *Journal of Clinical and Experimental Neuropsychology, 23*, 705–717.

Babikian, T., & Asarnow, R. (2009). Neurocognitive outcomes and recovery after pediatric TBI: Meta-analytic review of the literature. *Neuropsychology, 23*, 283–296.

Bernstein J.H., Waber D.P. (1990). Developmental neuropsychological assessment. In: Boulton A.A., Baker G.B., Hiscock M. (Eds.) Neuropsychology: Vol. 17. Neuromethods. Clifton NJ:Humana Press.

Bieri, D., Reeve, R., Champion, G. D., et al. (1990). The faces pain scale for the self-assessment of the severity of pain experienced by children: development, initial validation and preliminary investigation for ratio scale properties. *Pain, 41*, 139–150.

Camiolo Reddy, C., Collins, M. W., & Gioia, G. A. (2008). Adolescent sports concussion. *Physical Medicine and Rehabilitation Clinics of North America, 19*, 247–269.

Catroppa, C., Anderson, V., Morse, S., et al. (2007). Children's attentional skills 5 years post-TBI. *Journal of Pediatric Psychology, 32*, 354–369.

Centers for Disease Control and Prevention (CDC) (2007). National Center for Injury Prevention and Control. Heads Up: Brain Injury in your Practice. Facts for Physicians. Atlanta, Center for Disease Control and Prevention. Available via http://www.cdc.gov/ncipc/tbi/Physicians_Tool_Kit.htm. Cited 1 Feb 2011.

Collie, A., Darby, D., & Maruff, P. (2001). Computerized cognitive assessment of athletes with sports related head injury. *British Journal of Sports Medicine, 35*, 297–302.

Collie, A., & Maruff, P. (2003). Computerized cognitive assessment of concussed Australian Rules footballers. *British Journal of Sports Medicine, 37*, 2–3.

Collins, M. W., Lovell, M. R., Iverson, G. L., et al. (2002). Cumulative effects of concussion in high school athletes. *Neurosurgery, 51*, 1175–1179.

Collins, M. W., Lovell, M. R., Iverson, G. L., et al. (2006). Examining concussion rates and return to play in high school football players wearing newer helmet technology: a three year prospective cohort study. *Neurosurgery, 58*, 275–283.

Collins, M. W., Lovell, M. R., & McKeag, D. B. (1999). Current issues in managing sports-related concussion. *Journal of the American Medical Association, 282*, 2283–2285.

Comper, P., Bisschop, S. M., Carnide, N., et al. (2005). A systematic review of treatments for mild traumatic brain injury. *Brain Injury, 19*, 863–880.

De Los Reyes, A., & Kazdin, A. E. (2005). Informant discrepancies in the assessment of childhood psychopathology: a critical review, theoretical framework and recommendations for further study. *Psychological Bulletin, 131*, 483–509.

Echemendia, R. J., & Julian, L. J. (2001). Mild traumatic brain injury in sports: Neuropsychology's contribution to a developing field. *Neuropsychology Review, 11*, 69–88.

Fay, T. B., Yeates, K. O., Taylor, H. G., et al. (2010). Cognitive reserve as a moderator of postconcussive symptoms in children with complicated and uncomplicated mild traumatic brain injury. *Journal of International Neuropsychological Society, 16*, 94–105.

Fay, T. B., Yeates, K. O., Wade, S. L., et al. (2009). Predicting longitudinal patterns of functional deficits in children with traumatic brain injury. *Neuropsychology, 23*, 271–282.

Fazio, V. C., Lovell, M. R., Pardini, J. E., et al. (2007). The relation between post concussion symptoms and neurocognitive performance in concussed athletes. *NeuroRehabilitation, 22*, 207–216.

Field, M., Lovell, M. W., Collins, M. R., et al. (2003). Does age play a role in recovery from sports-related concussion? A comparison of high school and collegiate athletes. *The Journal of Pediatrics, 142*, 546–553.

Fritz, G. K., Yeung, A., Wamboldt, M. Z., et al. (1996). Conceptual and methodologic issues in quantifying perceptual accuracy in childhood asthma. *Journal of Pediatric Psychology, 21*, 153–173.

Frommer, L. J., Gurka, K. K., Cross, K. M., et al. (2011). Sex differences in concussion symptoms of high school athletes. *Journal of Athletic Training, 46*, 76–84.

Gagnon, I., Swaine, B., Friedman, D., et al. (2004). Children demonstrate decreased dynamic balance following a mild traumatic brain injury. *Archives of Physical Medicine and Rehabilitation, 85*, 444–452.

Gioia, G. A., Collins, M. W., & Isquith, P. K. (2008a). Improving identification and diagnosis of mild TBI with evidence: Psychometric support for the Acute Concussion Evaluation (ACE). *The Journal of Head Trauma Rehabilitation, 23*, 230–242.

Gioia, G. A., Isquith, P. K., Schneider, J. C., et al. (2009a). Initial validation of a pediatric version of the Immediate Post Concussion Assessment and Cognitive Testing (ImPACT) Battery [Abstract]. *British Journal of Sports Medicine, 43*(Suppl 1), i92.

Gioia, G. A., Janusz, J. A., Isquith, P. K., et al. (2008b). Psychometric properties of the parent and teacher post-concussion symptom inventory (PCSI) for children and adolescents. *Journal of International Neuropsychological Society, 14*(Suppl. 1), 204.

Gioia, G. A., Schneider, J. C., Vaughan, C. G., et al. (2009b). Which symptom assessments and approaches are uniquely appropriate for paediatric concussion. *British Journal of Sports Medicine, 43*(Suppl I), 13–22.

Gioia, G. A., Vaughan, C. G., & Isquith, P. K. (2011). *Manual for pediatric immediate post-concussion assessment and cognitive testing*. Pittsburgh, PA: ImPACT Applications, Inc.

Giza, C., & Prins, M. L. (2006). Is being plastic fantastic? Mechanisms of altered plasticity after developmental TBI. *Developmental Neuroscience, 28*, 364–379.

Guskiewicz, K. M., Perrin, D. H., & Gansneder, B. M. (1996). Effect of mild head injury on postural stability in athletes. *Journal of Athletic Training, 31*, 300–306.

Guskiewicz, K. M., Ross, S. E., & Marshall, S. W. (2001). Postural stability and neuropsychological deficits after concussion in collegiate athletes. *Journal of Athletic Training, 36*, 263–273.

Hajek, C. A., Yeates, K. O., Taylor, H. G., et al. (2011). Agreement between parents and children on ratings of post-concussive symptoms following mild traumatic brain injury. *Child Neuropsychology, 17*, 17–33.

Halstead, M. E., & Walter, K. D. (2010). Sport-related concussion in children and adolescents. *Pediatrics, 126*, 597–615.

Hawley, C. A., Ward, A. B., Magnay, A. R., et al. (2003). Parental stress and burden following traumatic brain injury amongst children and adolescents. *Brain Injury, 17*, 1–23.

Hessen, E., Nestvold, K., & Sundet, K. (2006). Neuropsychological function in a group of patients 25 years after sustaining minor head injuries as children and adolescents. *Scandinavian Journal of Psychology, 47*, 245–251.

Iverson, G. L., Brooks, B. L., Collins, M. W., et al. (2006). Tracking neuropsychological recovery following concussion in sport. *Brain Injury, 20*, 245–252.

Kirkwood, M. W., Yeates, K. O., Taylor, H. G., et al. (2008). Management of pediatric mild traumatic brain injury: a neuropsychological review from injury through recovery. *Clinical Neuropsychology, 22*, 769–800.

Kirkwood, M. W., Yeates, K. O., & Wilson, P. E. (2006). Pediatric sport-related concussion: a review of the clinical management of an oft-neglected population. *Pediatrics, 117*, 1359–1371.

Light, R., Asarnow, R. F., Satz, P., et al. (1998). Mild closed-head injury in children and adolescents: behavior problems and academic outcomes. *Journal of Consulting and Clinical Psychology, 66*, 1023–1029.

Lovell, M. R. (2008). The neurophysiology and assessment of sports-related head injuries. *Neurologic Clinics, 26*, 45–62.

Lovell, M. R., Collins, M. W., Iverson, G. L., et al. (2003). Recovery from mild concussion in high school athletes. *Journal of Neurosurgery, 98*, 295–301.

Lovell M, Collins M, Maroon J (2002). ImPACT: The best approach to concussion management, Version 2.1 User's Manual. Pittsburgh PA: Impact Test.

Lovell, M. R., & Fazio, V. (2008). Concussion management in the child and adolescent athlete. *Current Sports Medicine Reports, 7*, 12–15.

Lovell, M. R., Iverson, G. L., Collins, M. W., et al. (2006). Measurement of symptoms following sport-related concussion: reliability and normative data for the post-concussion scale. *Applied Neuropsychology, 13*, 166–174.

Mainwaring, L. M., Bisschop, S. M., Green, R. E., et al. (2004). Emotional reaction of varsity athletes to sport-related concussion. *Journal of Sport and Exercise Psychology, 26*, 119–135.

Majerske, C. W., Mihalik, J. P., Ren, D., et al. (2008). Concussion in sports: postconcussive activity levels, symptoms, and neurocognitive performance. *Journal of Athletic Training, 43*, 265–274.

Maroon, J. R., Lovell, M. R., Norwig, J., et al. (2000). Cerebral concussion in athletes: evaluation and neuropsychological testing. *Neurosurgery, 47*, 659–669.

Massagli, T. L., Fann, J. R., Burington, B. E., et al. (2004). Psychiatric illness after mild traumatic brain injury in children. *Archives of Physical Medicine and Rehabilitation, 85*, 1428–1434.

McCrea, M. (2008). *Mild traumatic brain injury and postconcussion syndrome*. New York: Oxford University Press.

McCrea, M., Barr, W. B., Guskiewicz, K., et al. (2005). Standard regression-based methods for measuring recovery after sports-related concussion. *Journal of International Neuropsychological Society, 11*, 58–69.

McCrea, M., Hammeke, T. A., Olsen, G., et al. (2004). Unreported concussion in high school football players: implications for prevention. *Clinical Journal of Sport Medicine, 14*, 13–17.

McCrory, P., Makdissi, M., Davis, G., et al. (2005). Value of neuropsychological testing after head injuries in football. *British Journal of Sports Medicine, 39*(Suppl), 58–63.

McKinlay, A., Dalrymple-Alford, J. C., Horwood, L. J., et al. (2002). Long term psychosocial outcomes after mild head injury in early childhood. *Journal of Neurology, Neurosurgery, and Psychiatry, 73*, 281–288.

Mihalik, J. P., Stump, J. E., Collins, M. W., et al. (2005). Posttraumatic migraine characteristics in athletes following sports-related concussion. *Journal of Neurosurgery, 102*, 850–855.

Moser, R. S., Schatz, P., & Jordan, B. D. (2005). Prolonged effects of concussion in high school athletes. *Neurosurgery, 57*, 300–306.

Pellman, E. J., Lovell, M. R., Viano, D. C., et al. (2006). Concussion in professional football: recovery in NFL and high school athletes assessed by computerized neuropsychological testing. *Neurosurgery, 58*, 263–274.

Ponsford, J., Willmott, C., Rothwell, A., et al. (1999). Cognitive and behavioral outcome following mild traumatic head injury in children. *The Journal of Head Trauma Rehabilitation, 14*, 360–372.

Ponsford, J., Willmott, C., Rothwell, A., et al. (2001). Impact of early intervention on outcome after mild traumatic brain injury in children. *Pediatrics, 108*, 1297–1303.

Riemann, B. L., & Guskiewicz, K. M. (2000). Effects of mild head injury on postural stability as measured through clinical balance testing. *Journal of Athletic Training, 35*, 19–25.

Riemann, B. L., Guskiewicz, K. M., & Shields, E. W. (1999). Relationship between clinical and forceplate measures of postural stability. *Journal of Sport Rehabilitation, 8*, 71–82.

Satz, P., Zaucha, K., McCleary, C., et al. (1997). Mild head injury in children and adolescents: a review of studies (1970–1995). *Psychological Bulletin, 122*, 107–131.

Schatz, P., Pardini, J. E., Lovell, M. R., et al. (2006). Sensitivity and specificity of the ImPACT test battery for concussion in athletes. *Archives of Clinical Neuropsychology, 21*, 91–99.

Swaine, B. R., Tremblay, C., Platt, R. W., et al. (2007). Previous head injury is a risk factor for subsequent head injury in children: a longitudinal cohort study. *Pediatrics, 119*, 749–758.

Taylor, H. G., Dietrich, A., Nuss, K., et al. (2010). Post-concussive symptoms in children with mild traumatic brain injury. *Neuropsychology, 24*, 148–159.

Turkstra, L. S., Coelho, C., & Ylvisaker, M. (2005). The use of standardized tests for individuals with cognitive-communication disorders. *Seminars in Speech and Language, 26*, 215–222.

Upton, P., Lawford, J., & Eiser, C. (2008). Parent-child agreement across child health-related quality of life instruments: a review of the literature. *Quality of Life Research, 17*, 895–913.

van Kampen, D. A., Lovell, M. R., Pardini, J. E., et al. (2006). The "value added" of neurocognitive testing after sports-related concussion. *The American Journal of Sports Medicine, 34*(10), 1630–1635.

Varni, J. W., Limbers, C. A., & Burwinkle, T. M. (2007a). How young can children reliably and validly self-report their health-related quality of life?: An analysis of 8,591 children across age subgroups with the PedsQL™ 4.0 generic core scales. *Health and Quality of Life Outcomes, 5*, 1.

Varni, J. W., Limbers, C. A., & Burwinkle, T. M. (2007b). Parent proxy-report of their children's health-related quality of life: An analysis of 13,878 parents' reliability and validity across age subgroups using the PedsQL™ 4.0 Generic Core Scales. *Health and Quality of Life Outcomes, 5*, 2.

Chapter 13
The Future of Preventing Concussion in Children and Adolescents

Rebecca A. Demorest

13.1 Introduction

Prevention of injury is one of the primary goals when it comes to youth participation in sports. Unfortunately, prevention of youth concussions is not particularly easy. Whether there has been an actual increase in the number of youth concussions, or just more recognition of concussion injuries, concussions are a concern for just about anyone playing sports. Knowledge regarding concussion mechanisms, consequences, management, and treatment is extremely important, but prevention should be the utmost goal. Research is sparse regarding how to adequately prevent concussions and available equipment is lacking in this protection. Most research is done at a collegiate or professional level making extrapolation of data to younger athletes, who may be more vulnerable to injury and have different mechanics, injury patterns and recovery, very challenging (McCrory et al. 2004; Lovell and Fazio 2008). Recognition and education regarding concussions is currently our best tool regarding avoidance of this devastating injury. This chapter will review the current research regarding principles of head injury as it may relate to prevention, current protective equipment and future insights into how to prevent concussion.

13.2 Principles of Head Injury as it Relates to Prevention of Concussion

Understanding the forces and parameters associated with head injury is the first step in trying to develop head and neck protection that may one day be able to prevent concussions.

R.A. Demorest (✉)
Associate Medical Director, Pediatric and Young Adult Sports Medicine,
Children's Hospital & Research Center Oakland, Oakland, CA, USA
e-mail: rebeccademorest@gmail.com

J.N. Apps and K.D. Walter (eds.), *Pediatric and Adolescent Concussion:*
Diagnosis, Management and Outcomes, DOI 10.1007/978-0-387-89545-1_13,
© Springer Science+Business Media, LLC 2012

Current research suggests that there is debate over the most meaningful biomechanical factors associated with head injury; acceleration (translational/linear vs. rotational), the relative changes in velocity and impact speed during head impact, and head displacement. Newer research is focusing on which of these parameters is paramount in being responsible for the clinical changes seen with concussion so that this information may be used to better equip athletes with risk reducing equipment when possible.

13.2.1   Biomechanics of Football Head Impacts

Most current clinical research regarding biomechanical forces associated with head injury, as it relates to concussion, is performed through the professional National Football League (NFL). In 1994, the NFL formed a committee through which mild traumatic brain injuries (mTBIs) are currently being studied (Pellman 2003). These research efforts evaluate game videos of NFL concussions followed by laboratory reconstructions of those impacts in order to further evaluate the forces associated with head impact. For full information regarding NFL protocol and study parameters please (see Pellman et al. 2003a). There are a few studies at the collegiate football level and even fewer at the high school and pee-wee football level, making extrapolation of data to the pediatric and adolescent age level challenging. Head injury research in other sports including ice hockey, boxing and soccer is also paramount in recognizing the biomechanics of concussions, although most research is again, not at a true pediatric or adolescent level, focusing rather on collegiate, amateur or professional athletes.

13.2.1.1   Football Head Impact Kinematics

NFL data suggests that with NFL football head impacts, initial head impact occurs over 10 milliseconds (ms) (Pellman et al. 2003b). Impact forces peak at 6-8ms with forces and head accelerations declining by 10ms (Pellman et al. 2003b). Rapid head displacement occurs over 20ms; with head displacement and rotation occurring at 10-20ms, and neck compressive forces at 20ms (Pellman et al. 2003b). This information may be helpful in delineating which forces are truly associated with clinical concussion symptoms which may then translate into how to provide protection against these forces with equipment modification.

13.2.1.2   Peak Translational Acceleration

Peak translational (linear) acceleration of the head is one force that is thought to be directly responsible for concussion. Studies at various levels differ as to what threshold of translational acceleration is required to cause a clinical concussion. It can be difficult to extrapolate this data to the pediatric level as pediatric brains differ from adult brains.

Average football peak acceleration of head impacts in those not sustaining a concussion varies. In a study of 132 impacts, occurring in 2 high school football players, the average peak acceleration sustained by non-concussive forces was 29.2 grams (g) (Naunheim et al. 2000). Collegiate studies report average non-concussive forces of 20.1 g +/− 18.7 g (n=11601 impacts) (Brolinson et al. 2006) and 32 g +/−25 g (n=3312 impacts) (Duma et al. 2005). In one study of Division I football, non-concussion acceleration impacts for collegiate lineman ranged from 20–23 g (Mihalik et al. 2007). The average peak acceleration in NFL players not sustaining a concussion was 60g +/− 24 g (n=31) (Pellman et al. 2003a). The fact that the NFL data supports a much higher average peak acceleration for non-concussion impacts compared with collegiate and high school studies needs to be taken with concern when using this data to extrapolate to a younger age group.

Similarly, average peak translational acceleration of head impacts in those sustaining a concussion also varies. The NFL reported an average peak acceleration of 98 g +/− 28 g in those with a concussion (n=31) (Pellman et al. 2003a) versus 81 g in college (n=1) (Duma et al. 2005). NFL findings suggest that concussions are primarily related to translational head acceleration (Pellman et al. 2003a). One study showed that college players underwent high level impacts (>98 g) more frequently than high school players (Schnebel et al. 2007). A rugby study of unhelmeted concussive head injuries, evaluated through numerical reconstructions of video footage, showed an average peak linear acceleration of 86 g (Frechede and McIntosh 2009). Again, extrapolation to the pediatric age group needs to be further evaluated and taken with concern. It appears that younger athletes may not undertake as many high level hits as older athletes, but how this relates to their risk for concussion has yet to be determined, as it may take less of a force to cause a concussion sustaining impact in this young group.

Trends suggest that professional football athletes may have harder concussive and non-concussive head hits along with a higher threshold for sustaining a concussion. Variations in study methods and reporting severity may account for some of these differences. The NFL studies selected more severe open field hits and used hybrid dummies for reconstructions of concussive impacts after evaluation of video data whereas the collegiate studies evaluated true on field hits through a helmet accelerometer system. There is also the suggestion that real head impacts may be more severe than laboratory reconstructions which may distort the data (Frechede and McIntosh 2009; McIntosh and McCrory 2000).

13.2.1.3   Rotational Acceleration

Data from the boxing literature suggests that rotational acceleration may be the key force regarding severe head injury and potentially responsible for the chronic encephalopathy that is currently seen in boxers. Boxer head punches have lower translational but higher rotational acceleration than football head impacts

(Viano et al. 2005b). It is postulated that a more efficient transfer of energy may occur with translational acceleration that results in visible concussion symptoms (Viano et al. 2005b). These symptoms may cause an athlete to be taken out of play earlier versus a boxer with less translational but more rotational forces, who may play for longer and sustain further injury while impaired (Viano et al. 2005b). These rotational forces may be detrimental over time. Rotational acceleration and how it relates to concussions is being investigated in current football research.

13.2.1.4 Relative Changes in Head Impact Velocity, Impact Speed, and Duration

Changes in head velocity, impact speed and impact duration are currently under evaluation in terms of how they impact concussion injury. In the NFL, concussion impacts have been shown to have an average impact speed of 20.8 +/− 4.2 miles/hour (9.3 m/s), a change in head velocity of 16.1 mph (7.2 m/s), and a 98g head acceleration of 15 ms with strikes being oblique to the facemask, facemask attachment or to the side of the helmet (Pellman et al. 2003a). Mean change in velocity for rugby concussions was 4 m/s (McIntosh et al. 2000). Non-concussed NFL football players showed average impact speeds of 11.2+/− 2.5 miles/h (Pellman et al. 2003a).

A rapid change in head velocity is thought to lead to head displacement which may be a key factor in brain injury (Denny-Brown and Russell 1941). Some NFL studies suggest that changes in velocity may be more significant than acceleration in determining concussion thresholds (Pellman et al. 2003b; Viano et al. 2007).

The 15 millisecond duration of impact seen in NFL concussions is much longer than the typical impact associated with car crashes (< 6 ms) (Pellman et al. 2003a). The highest brain strains occur more than 10ms after high impact forces with the greatest rates of strain seen in the midbrain, fornix and corpus collosum (Viano et al. 2005a). These strained areas may correlate with certain symptoms experienced during a concussion (cognitive and memory problems, loss of consciousness, and inability to return to play) (Viano et al. 2005a). This information may help to assist researchers in developing equipment best suited to help prevent clinical concussions and limit their symptoms.

13.2.2 Location of Football Head Impacts and Risk Associated with Player Position and Plays

Oblique and side hits to the facemask area in football seem to be a vulnerable area for concussion. In studied NFL concussive impacts, 61% of impacts were helmet to helmet, usually oblique strikes to the facemask, 16% were shoulder pads to head and 16% were caused by ground impact (Pellman et al. 2003a). Greater than 50% of concussive impacts in the NFL involved the facemask or facemask attachment area to the helmet for the struck player (Pellman et al. 2003a). The majority of rugby concussion occurring impacts were to the temporal region with 86% occurring to the anterior half of head, 10% to the occipital region and 3% to the upper body (McIntosh et al. 2000). These studies support the idea that side blows to the face-mask and temporal regions of the skull may be responsible for the majority of concussions. Developing equipment to protect the head from these blows, if possible, is the next step.

In the NFL, risk for concussion was highest for quarterbacks (1.62 concussions/100 game positions (GP)), wide receivers (1.23/100GP), tight ends (.94/100GP) and the defensive secondary (.93/100GP) (Viano et al. 2007). Also in the NFL, the riskiest plays for concussions were kickoff (9.29 concussions /1000 plays), punts (3.86/1000 plays), rushing (2.24/1000 plays) and passing plays (2.14/1000 plays) (Viano et al. 2007).

In a Division 1 collegiate study, football offensive lineman sustained the greatest number of head impacts with their average non-concussed acceleration impacts ranging from 20–23 g (Mihalik et al. 2007) 18.81% of impacts occurred to the top of the head (Mihalik et al. 2007). Acceleration impacts in helmets-only full contact practices were higher than in games or scrimmages at the collegiate level (Mihalik et al. 2007), which is surprising as injury rates and possibly force, typically tend to be higher in games than in practices.

13.2.3 Can a Concussion Threshold be Established for Football?

Despite the above research, it is difficult to establish a true threshold for concussive injuries secondary to many contributing factors at many different levels, when it comes to concussions (Mihalik et al. 2007; Guskiewicz et al. 2007). According to NFL data, where the concussion threshold seems to be 70–75 g, 75% of impacts >98 g are expected to be concussive impacts (Pellman 2003a). This may or may not hold true for collegiate, high school or younger players and more research is needed before such a statement can be made.

One question that arises is how does the number of lower magnitude impacts received affect a possible threshold? Looking at collegiate data, skill position players seem to have a higher percentage of increased level impacts (60–98 g) versus lineman (Schnebel et al. 2007). Lineman, however, have the highest number of actual impacts but a low magnitude hit with almost every hit (20–30 g) (Schnebel et al. 2007). More research is needed to see what tolerance, if any occurs after repeated impacts and how cumulative effects, whether of concussion or non-concussion thresholds, will affect outcomes. Is there a higher risk for high school football athletes playing both ways secondary to the increased number and potential repeated exposures to sub-concussive hits? Further research will hopefully help to answer these questions.

13.2.4   Correlation of Football Head Impact with Concussion Symptoms

Although research can help determine magnitude, timing and changes in velocity and acceleration of impacts, how this clinically relates to concussions is the real question. Some studies suggest that linear impact forces may not necessarily correlate with clinical concussion symptoms (Guskiewicz et al. 2007; McCaffrey et al. 2007). In an NFL study, there was no immediate change in balance or cognition in NFL players after one exposure to a >90 g hit within 24 h (McCaffrey et al. 2007). One NFL study suggested that during a concussion, the greatest rates of strain seen in the midbrain, fornix and corpus collosum may correlate with clinical symptoms of cognitive and memory problems, loss of consciousness and inability to return to play (Viano et al. 2005a). More research is necessary in this area to determine how head impact forces, velocity, and timing correlate with physical or clinical symptoms and outcomes associated with concussions. It is only after that question is answered that a further in depth exploration of safety equipment to prevent concussions can be undertaken.

13.2.5   Soccer Concussions and Heading

Concussions from soccer seem to occur most often from contact with another player or another player's body part. Sixty-eight percent of soccer concussions in one study were a result of player collision (Barnes et al. 1998). In 29 soccer concussions occurring in 26 college players over 2 years, 0 were from heading; 28% were from contact with the player's head; 24% from impact with the ball; 14% from elbow contact; 10% from ground contact; and 6% from lower extremity contact (Boden et al. 1998). One study suggests that competing for head balls may increase the risk for head injury (Kirkendall et al. 2001).

Linear heading, by returning the soccer ball to the same direction in which it came, simulates a majority of game heading while rotational heading is used less frequently with heading in the penalty box. The peak acceleration from linearly headed balls approaches 49.3–54.7 g when kicked at 35–40 mph from 30 yards away (Naunheim et al. 2000; Lewis et al. 2001).

In purposeful heading of a soccer ball, the neck muscles forcibly contract to stabilize the head. This addition of mass from the neck and trunk lowers the ball mass to head ratio which may help to decrease impact forces compared with a ball hitting an unprepared head (Guskiewicz et al. 2002).

Questions have been raised as to whether the sub-concussive forces seen over time in soccer ball heading cause or contribute to chronic brain damage. Soccer players have been compared to boxers, with the concern that soccer athletes may also be at risk for chronic encephalopathy due to repeated head impacts. Earlier European studies supported this claim, but are judged as having faulty methods and not taking into effect co-founding factors such as age, alcohol intake, and previous head injury which could cause confusion in interpretation of results (Putukian et al. 2000).

Current prospective studies do not support the idea that heading causes acute impairment or chronic injury. One collegiate heading session did not lead to acute neuropsychological changes in cognitive function although practice effects and gender differences with certain tests were seen (Putukian et al. 2000). No acute changes in postural stability (balance-sensory interaction) with heading 20 balls at a fixed speed were seen in collegiate soccer athletes (Broglio et al. 2004). In another collegiate study, there was no association with cognitive decline, based on neuropsychological testing, in soccer athletes versus non-soccer athletes versus non-athletes; although soccer players did sustain more concussions than the other groups (Guskiewicz et al. 2002). In a study of 25 men of the US National Soccer team, there was no evidence that heading exposure correlated with symptoms attributable to chronic encephalopathy (Jordan et al. 1996). More studies, especially in the pediatric and adolescent age ranges need to be undertaken in order to explore the risks, if any, of soccer heading.

Some have suggested that the greatest injury risk in regards to heading may be in younger players who are not knowledgeable in proper heading technique. Proper heading technique, paying attention to the game, and playing with skillful players may be the best protection (Broglio et al. 2004). Using newer balls may also help to decrease injury risk as old leather balls tend to absorb water and can increase in weight by 20% when fully saturated (Delaney and Drummond 1999). Newer balls maintain constant weight and may afford a decreased risk of injury (Delaney and Drummond 1999).

13.3   Protective Equipment

13.3.1   Football Helmets

Initially made of leather, the first documented use of a football helmet was in the 1893 Army-Navy game (Levy et al. 2004b). Helmet use became mandatory for the NCAA in 1939 and the NFL in 1940 (Levy et al. 2004b). In 1969, the National Operating Committee on Standards for Athletic Equipment (NOCSAE) began research efforts for the first safety standards for helmets which were implemented in 1973 and accepted by the NCAA in 1978 and the National Federation of State High School Associations in 1980 (NFSHSA) (Hodgson 1975). All current helmets for high school and college need to be certified to the NOCSAE standard.

No previous or current football helmet has been shown to prevent a concussion. Initial helmets were designed to reduce the risk of skull fractures. In the 1970s, improvements to the football helmet including thick padded liners, 4 way chin straps, smoother outer shells and a change from web suspension to internal padding in order to try to lengthen the duration of impact and reduce the frequency of skull fractures and concussions (Viano et al. 2007). NOCSAE testing calculates a Severity

Index (SI) with current limits of 1200 for NOCSAE approved helmets. According the NOCSAE instruction manual "a headgear is positioned on a headform and then dropped in order to achieve an accepted impact velocity within 3% of the theoretical free fall velocity for that drop height. At impact, the instantaneous resultant acceleration is measured by the triaxial accelerometer and the Severity Index calculated." (NOCSAE 2010). NFL studies by Pellman suggest an SI threshold of 300 to prevent NFL concussion (Pellman et al. 2003a). No information is available regarding what threshold, if any, is suitable to prevent concussions in youth athletes.

Significant reduction in head and neck injuries occurred with the voluntary use of NOCSAE standards and rule changes. An increase in football neck and spine injuries from 1965–1975 resulted in rule changes that prohibited spearing, using the head and neck as a battling weapon (see Rule section 13.4). These rule changes resulted in a significant decrease in overall head and neck injuries (Levy et al. 2004b). NOCSAE standards also helped to decrease football fatalities by 74% and serious head injuries decreased from 4.25 per 100,000 to .68/100,000 (Levy et al. 2004a, b. Youth football had a 51% reduction in fatal head injuries, 35% reduction in concussions and 65% reduction in cranial fractures (Hodgson 1980).

Helmets and current NOCSAE testing support protection of head areas from linear impact only. NOCSAE testing drops a headform on a rigid anvil to determine linear impact. No rotational assessment is done, which may be more indicative of concussion in newer studies (Pellman et al. 2003a). Testing is also done primarily to impacts to the periphery or crown of the helmet. As some studies suggest that the majority of impact forces occur to the facemasks at oblique or lateral angles, this testing may not evaluate these types of hits (Pellman et al. 2003a). New testing is being developed with a pendulum to try to account for rotational effects.

13.3.2 New Helmet Design

Preliminary NFL evidence suggests that newer helmets might decrease but not prevent concussions. In 2000, new helmet design arose (Adams USA Pro Elite, Riddell Revolution, Schutt Sport Air Varsity Commander and DNA) which at the NFL level showed a 10% reduction in peak head acceleration and up to a 20% reduction in rotational acceleration (Viano et al. 2006) but have not yet been correlated with concussion risk.

Riddell's Revolution was the first helmet to come out of this testing in January 2002 (Pellman et al. 2006). The Revolution helmet was designed to reduce impact forces from blows to the side of the head and face (Collins et al. 2006). The helmet design has an exterior shell that extends anterior and distal to the traditional shell shape along the mandible; has an increased offset from the interior surface of the shell to the wearer's head, a unique interior liner construction and a new padded area over the zygoma and lateral parts of the mandible for side head and face blows (Collins et al. 2006).

In a 3 year study of 136 concussions in 2141 high school players wearing Revolution vs. standard helmets, a 31% decrease in relative risk and a 2.3% absolute risk reduction for sustaining a concussion was seen in athletes wearing Revolution helmets (Collins et al. 2006). Bias in this study includes a small number of concussed athletes, differences in age between the two groups (the Revolution group was approximately 6 months older than the standard group, so if younger athletes are more prone to concussions this could create bias), non-randomization of helmet type to player and no mention of the age of the standard helmets leading to possible non-acceptable helmets being used. There were no differences in on the field concussion markers, immediate symptoms, method of contact, location of head strike, or recovery rates between the groups. Custom helmets, such as the Xeneth are currently being marketed, but again no conclusive evidence suggests that they prevent concussions. Further study is needed to evaluate the effects these newer helmets may have on decreasing concussion risk.

13.3.3 Thoughts for Future Football Helmet Design

Although there is currently not a football helmet that prevents concussions, research regarding design may be promising. Studies have shown that many concussions cause early strains to the temporal and orbital-frontal complex lobe causing dizziness with later strains secondary to rotational forces to the fornix, midbrain and corpus callosum which correlates with memory and cognitive function and removal from play after concussion (Viano et al. 2005a). This knowledge may help with helmet design.

Increasing helmet thickness and energy absorption properties of the padding along with changes to the sides and backs of helmets may help reduce forces (Viano et al. 2006). An increase in energy absorbing padding decreased head accelerations over older helmet design in NFL players (Pellman et al. 2006). Decreasing the stiffness in the top and crown of the helmet, which tends to be stiffer than the sides, may help to decrease the forces seen when the striking player's crown hits the struck player's helmet sides (Viano and Pellman 2005). Reducing the mass of the helmet to lower the inertia of the striking player during impact may also help to reduce impact forces (Viano and Pellman 2005).

Limiting head movement after impact to reduce rotational forces is also encouraging. Impacts to facemasks resulted in larger head rotations than impacts to the helmet shell (Viano et al. 2007). These impacts, along with impacts to the chin are further from the head axis with a greater moment arm causing greater rotational displacement (Viano et al. 2007). Newer ideas to change the design of facemasks and chinstraps may help to stop this displacement (Viano et al. 2007).

Research can help to improve design; however simple fit and correct application of the helmet is of utmost importance if helmets are expected to reduce injury risk. In a study of Wisconsin high school football athletes, 84% did not have a football helmet that fit them correctly, with freshman having more fitting errors than seniors

(McGuine and Nass 1996). Underinflation of the bladder and using helmets that are old, too big or too small, may be the real concern in younger players, as money for the "newest helmet" does not always trickle down to that level. Information regarding how to properly fit a football helmet may be accessed at http://www.osaa.org/football/sportsmedicine/FittingFootballHelmets.pdf (cited on 4/29/10).

13.3.4   Soccer Headgear- Does it Decrease the Risk for Concussion?

Soccer headgear has been marketed to help reduce the impact associated with heading and head hits and ultimately the risk for concussion. Research is sparse and results are inconclusive but tend to support the idea that soccer headgear does not decrease the risk of concussion.

An adolescent retrospective study, with flaws, (the headgear group had a higher rate of previous concussions and 4 out of 5 athletes did not know they had had a concussion) suggested that those wearing headgear and females had a decreased risk of concussions (Delaney et al. 2008). One study suggests that headgear was not effective at reducing the impact from heading and high speed ball impact, but did offer some protection against impact from another player's head contact, whether voluntary or incidental (Withnall et al. 2005).

Concerns regarding soccer headgear as harmful exist due to possible increased rotational forces to the head and an increased risk for a more aggressive style of play while wearing a headgear (Guskiewicz et al. 2002; Withnall et al. 2005). With ball impact, because the human head is stiffer than the soccer ball, the ball deforms more than the head leading to increased energy and forces being transmitted to the head (Withnall et al. 2005). Typical sports head protection (helmets) affords a soft sacrificial (weak) layer that absorbs this force during impact, decreasing the energy, force and acceleration to the head (Withnall et al. 2005). In one study evaluating headgear while heading (using non-human test models), the amount of ball deformation during a heading scenario, was nearly ten times greater than the thickness of the headgear being used thereby affording no protection to the head (Withnall et al. 2005). Because the stiffness and deformation of the two objects (head and soccer ball) are largely different, the headgear was not effective in dissipating the forces. Headgear design would need to provide extremely thick and/or softer headbands to help dissipate the forces (Withnall el al. 2005). This design may result in poor athlete acceptance and ability in heading and controlling the ball (Withnall et al. 2005).

13.3.5   Other Sport Headgear

Ice hockey and rugby headgear have also been tested to see if improvements and/or use reduce the risk for concussion. Full and partial face masks reduced eye and face injuries and did not increase neck injuries or concussion (Stuart et al. 2002). Use of full faceguards in University hockey players reduced the number of games missed but not the incidence of concussion compared with half faceguards (Benson et al. 2002). Thicker rugby headgear may decrease impact attenuation (McIntosh et al. 2004). In a study of 13–20 year old male rugby players, there was no decrease in head injury or concussion in those using padded headgear although compliance was low (McIntosh et al. 2009). More research is necessary in all sports regarding head injury, protection, and concussion risk.

13.3.6   Mouthguards and Concussions

It has been suggested that mouthguards decrease the risk of concussion in athletes. There are no conclusive studies to date that prove that use of mouthguards decreases the risk of concussions, although they may decrease the risk of mouth and dental trauma (DeSmarteau 2006).

Mouthguards were mandated for use in high school football in 1962 and in the NCAA in 1974. There are 3 different types of mouthgards for athletic use; stock, boil and bite, and custom. Boil and bite mouthguards have the athlete heat the plastic mouthguard and bite to form an impression. The problem with these mouthguards is that biting pressure is hard to control so that posterior occlusal thickness, which is the protective quality, may be less than adequate. Custom mouthguards are either vacuum formed or pressure laminated. These allow greater control for posterior thickness, which is ideally 3-4mm and show little deformation over time (DeSmarteau 2006).

Potential benefits to mouthguard use include dissipation of forces to the maxilla, skull and temporomandibular joint (TMJ) when the mandible receives blows; stabilization of the skull though clenching which increases neck muscle activity; and a proper mandible position distracting the condyle from the fossa (Takeda 2005). In artificial skull models, distortion of the mandibular bone and acceleration of the head were decreased in those wearing a mouthguard (Takeda 2005).

One high school study with a low sample size (n=28) and most athletes having previous concussions, suggested that custom mouthguards may help decrease the risk of concussions in high school football athletes (Singh et al. 2009). One study showed no change in concussion rates with different mouthguard designs (Barbic and Brison 2005). There was no difference in concussions between custom and non-custom mouthguard use in Division I football (Wisniewski et al. 2004). Custom mouthguards (n = 8663 exposures) did not decrease the rate of oral soft tissue injury or concussion in Division I men's NCAA basketball but did reduce the risk of dental injuries (LaBella et al. 2002).

Design concerns regarding mouthgard studies include no quality standards of those mouthguards being studied, with concern that some mouthguards may be altered to fit by athletes, causing a reduction of the protective qualities. Removal of the posterior tooth coverage decreases protective coverage but is common practice among users of boil and bite mouthguards for comfort reasons. No study has evaluated the fit of mouthguards followed by whether or not they help reduce the risk of concussions.

Most concussions, secondary to mechanism, may not be able to be prevented with use of a mouthguard. One study found that only 1.6% of concussions occurred with a blow to the jaw while 61.2 % occurred with head to head contact (Wisniewski et al. 2004). There may also be a difference in protection afforded by mouthguards depending on whether the sport uses a helmet (football) versus no helmet (basketball). More research is needed in this field.

13.3.7   Other Equipment and Environmental Factors

Other equipment or environmental factors may contribute to concussion risk. The hardness of the ground my allow athletes to move faster thus causing more force with hits (McIntosh and McCrory 2005). One study supported the idea that artificial surfaces may contribute to concussions (Naunheim et al. 2002). Using appropriate sized soccer balls that do not retain water and are not hyperinflated along with padded soccer goalposts may help to decrease injury risk.

13.4   Will Rule Changes Prevent Concussions?

Between 1971–73, 39% of quadriplegia from football resulted from axial loading (direct linear compression of head and neck in parallel with the cervical spine) mechanisms (Torg 1991). The no "spearing" rule, instituted by the NCAA and NFL at the end of the 1975 season, was created secondary to an increase in the number of head and neck injuries that were occurring in football. As the majority of cervical fractures and dislocations are caused by axial loading, rule changes in football banning deliberate spearing (intentional head down striking of a player with the top or crown of the helmet (Levy et al. 2004a) decreased severe cervical spine injuries in the 1970s with continued decline in the following decades (Heck et al. 2004).

Striking players line up the head, neck, and torso in order to deliver maximum force in NFL helmet to helmet impacts. Helmet impacts are 61% of concussive collisions in the NFL (Viano and Pellman 2005). To ensure delivery of momentum to the struck player, the striking player maintains axial alignment, minimizes neck extension and lateral bending, and engages the helmet of the struck player. A concussive blow in the head down position increases momentum by increasing the mass of the striking player by 67% through engagement of his torso in the blow (Viano and Pellman 2005). If the struck player is able to anticipate the hit, he can line up his torso and resist the impact by leaning into the tackle and lining up his body; however the struck player does not usually see the hit coming. A heads- up stance reduces collision inertial load and impact forces and could decrease the risk of concussion in a struck player (Viano and Pellman 2005).

Striking players, along with struck players, however, are at risk for injury during spearing and axial load mechanisms. The average peak neck compressive force is greater in striking players compared with struck players sustaining concussions suggesting an increased risk for cervical spine or spinal cord injuries in the striking athlete. The average peak head acceleration for a struck NFL concussed player is greatest at 94.3 g +/− 24.5 g versus 67.9 g +/− 14.5 for a non concussed struck player versus 56.1 g +/− 22.1 for a striking player using spearing (Viano and Pellman 2005). Striking players have lower forces because of added mass through neck compression. However as of a 2005 NFL study, no striking NFL player had sustained a serious neck injury probably because of a greater mass to withstand injury and stronger neck muscles (Viano and Pellman 2005).

A heads-up stance might also decrease the risk of neck injury in the striking player. If the mass of the struck player is substantial the impact load gets put back on the striking player (Viano and Pellman 2005). This causes the neck to buckle in flexion or lateral bending therefore increasing the risk of fracture, dislocation or spinal cord injury (Viano and Pellman 2005). Avoiding spearing and keeping a "heads up" tackling position may be even more important at the younger levels, where neck muscles are likely to be weaker and technique less standard.

Rules in other sports may help to decrease the risk for concussions. In Canadian amateur ice hockey, the greatest cause of concussion was contact with the ice or boards (Goodman et al. 2001). Illegal actions, such as elbowing, also caused concussions with >20% of concussions sustained from elbow contact to the jaw or another part of the head (Goodman et al. 2001). Body checking, especially from behind, has been associated with concussion risk (Pashby et al. 2001). Elimination of plays where the intent is to injure the other player are recommended to reduce the risk for concussion (Goodman et al. 2001). Elimination of head checking with any part of the body (head, elbow, shoulder) may be an effective way to decrease concussion (Biasca et al. 2002). In 2002, the International Ice Hockey Federation introduced a new rule to eliminate every "clean check" to the head (Biasca et al. 2002).

13.5 Does Neck Strengthening Prevent Concussions?

Some suggest that increased neck strength in flexion, extension, and lateral bending may help to decrease the risk for concussion. Neck compression forces of greater than 4000N are considered sufficient to seriously injure a player because of axial compression to the cervical spine (Viano and Pellman 2004). Increasing neck stiffness in dummies reduces the peak head acceleration and change in velocity so strengthening may be beneficial for controlling head responses and hence concussion risk (Viano et al. 2007). Children and females with weaker necks may have a disproportionate increase in head velocity which could increase the risk for concussion (Viano et al. 2007). It is postulated that kids may take longer to heal from concussions secondary to higher head displacement which causes higher strains in the midbrain with concussion (Viano et al. 2007). How much neck muscle strength contributes to reduction in concussion risk is still under investigation. It is difficult to isolate this one characteristic, as youth brain development, a complex and major contributing factor to head injury recovery, is under continued investigation.

13.6 Education and Recognition of Concussions

Education and awareness of concussion may be the best prevention tool that we currently have. In a study of 1532 high school football players, only 47.3% of athletes who sustained a concussion reported it to a coach or athletic trainer when it occurred (McCrea et al. 2004). The most common reasons for not reporting were not thinking it warranted medical attention (66.4%), not wanting to be withheld from competition (41%), and a lack of awareness of concussion (36.1%) (McCrea et al. 2004). A study of 461 University college athletes showed that 56% had no knowledge of consequences following a head injury; had a tendency to play while symptomatic (dizziness 28.2%, headache 30.4%, reporting a concussion 19.5%) and had a failure to report symptoms while playing (almost 20%) especially among football players (Kaut et al. 2003).

The theory of risk compensation, playing more aggressively secondary to the belief of a decreased risk for injury, also affects those using equipment to try to prevent concussions. Protective equipment may prompt players to act more aggressively and subsequently increase the risk of injury (Hagel and Meeuwisse 2004; McIntosh 2005). Sixty seven percent of rugby players wearing headgear felt more confident and felt they were able to tackle harder while wearing the headgear (Finch et al. 2001).

Recognition of risk factors (previous head injuries or concussions and continued cognitive deficits) through a proper pre-participation evaluation is promoted as a way to help prevent injury (McIntosh and McCrory 2005). Training of health professionals including physicians, nurses, physician assistants, EMTs, first responders, athletic trainers and coaches is also paramount to prevention and recognition of concussions. The CDC Tool Kit is a great educational resource for coaches, parents and athletes regarding concussions, risk, and prevention (http://www.cdc.gov/concussion/HeadsUp/youth.html accessed 3/14/10).

13.7 Conclusion

More research is necessary, especially in the pediatric and adolescent age groups, in regards to prevention of concussion. There is promising football research, especially at the collegiate and NFL level, regarding head impact kinematics and evaluation of concussive versus non-concussive hits that may help with future design of helmets and protective equipment. Although not proven to prevent concussions, football helmets and mouthgards are recommended for their known protective effects when appropriate. Soccer heading, in and of itself, has not been shown to cause acute concussive symptoms or chronic changes seen following repeated head injury. Following of rules and engaging in safe play is highly recommended to help prevent significant head injury. Recognition and education regarding concussions may be our best method of concussion prevention.

13.8   Key Points

Current research suggests that there is debate over the most meaningful biomechanical factors associated with head injury; acceleration (translational/linear vs. rotational), the relative changes in velocity and impact speed during head impact, and head displacement.

Hits to the facemask or temporal head region may be significant in causing concussion.

Soccer heading, in and of itself, has not been shown to cause concussion.

Football helmets, designed to protect against serious head and neck injury, have not been shown to prevent concussion although new research may be promising in this field.

Soccer headgear has not been shown to prevent concussion.

Mouthguards help protect against mouth and dental trauma, but have not been shown to prevent concussion.

Prohibiting football spearing, using the head and neck as a battling weapon, has helped to decrease severe cervical spine injuries.

Rule changes for safe play may be helpful in decreasing injury risk.

Neck strengthening may help decrease impact forces but has not conclusively been shown to prevent concussion.

Education and recognition are the best current methods for preventing and protecting youth athletes from concussions and their potentially devastating consequences.

Further research, especially in the pediatric and adolescent age group, is needed to further evaluate methods to prevent concussion.

References

Barbic D, Pater J, Brison RJ (2005) Comparison of mouth guard designs and concussion prevention in contact sports. *Clinical Journal of Sport Medicine, 15*, 294–298.

Barnes B, Cooper L, Kirkendall D. et al. (1998) Concussion History in elite male and female soccer players. *The American Journal of Sports Medicine, 26*, 433–438.

Benson BW, Rose MS, Meeuwisse WH (2002) The impact of face shield use on concussion in ice hockey: a multivariate analysis. *British Journal of Sports Medicine, 36*, 27–32.

Biasca N, Wirth S, Tegner Y (2002) The avoidability of head and neck injuries in ice hockey: an historical review. *British Journal of Sports Medicine, 36*, 410–427.

Boden B, Kirkendall D, Garrett W (1998) Concussion incidence in elite college soccer players. *The American Journal of Sports Medicine, 26*, 238–241.

Broglio SP, Guskiewicz KM, Sell TC, et al. (2004) No acute changes in postural control after soccer heading. *British Journal of Sports Medicine, 38*, 561–567.

Brolinson PG, Manoogian S, McNeely D, et al. (2006) Analysis of Linear Head Accelerations from Collegiate Football Impacts. *Current Sports Medicine Reports, 5*, 23–28.

Collins M, Lovell MR, Iverson GL, et al. (2006) Examining Concussion Rates and Return to Play in High School Football Players Wearing Newer Helmet Technology: A Three Year Prospective Cohort Study. *Neurosurgery, 58*, 275–286.

Delaney JS, Drummond R (1999) Has the Time come for protective headgear for soccer? *Clinical Journal of Sport Medicine, 9*, 121–123.

Delaney JS, Al-Kashmiri A, Drummond R et al. (2008) The effect of protective headgear on head injuries and concussions in adolescent football (Soccer) players. *British Journal of Sports Medicine, 42*, 110–115.

Denny-Brown D, Russell R (1941) Experimental Cerebral Concussion. *Brain, 64*, 7–164.

DeSmarteau D (2006) Recommendation for the use of mouthguards in contact sports: can they also reduce the incidence and severity of cerebral concussions? *Current Sports Medicine Reports, 5*, 268–271.

Duma SM, Manoogian SJ, Bussone WR, et al. (2005)Analysis of Real-time Head Accelerations in Collegiate Football Players. *Clinical Journal of Sport Medicine, 15*(1):3–8.

Finch CF, McIntosh AS, McCrory P (2001) What do under 15 year old school-boy rugby union players think about protective headgear? *British Journal of Sports Medicine, 35*, 89–94.

Frechede B. McIntosh AS (2009) Numerical Reconstruction of Real-Life Concussive Football Impacts. *Medicine and Science in Sports and Exercise, 41*(2): 390–398.

Goodman D, Gaetz M, Meichenbaum D (2001) Concussions in hockey: there is cause for concern. *Medicine and Science in Sports and Exercise, 33*(12): 2004–2009.

Guskiewicz KM, Marshall SW, Broglio SP, et al. (2002) No evidence of impaired neurocognitive performance in collegiate soccer players. *The American Journal of Sports Medicine, 30*(2): 157–162.

Guskiewicz KM, Mihalik JP, Shankar V. et al. (2007) Measurement of Head Impacts in Collegiate Football Players: Relationship Between Head Impact Biomechanics and Acute Clinical Outcome After Concussion. *Neurosurgery, 61*, 1244–1253.

Hagel B, Meeuwisse (2004) Risk Compensation: a side effect of sport injury prevention? *Clinical Journal of Sport Medicine, 14*(4): 193–196.

Heck JF. Clarke KS, Peterson TR et al. (2004) National Athletic Trainer's Association Position Statement: Head-down contact and spearing in tackle football. *Journal of Athletic Training, 39*, 101–111.

Hodgson VR (1975) National Operating Committee on Standards for Athletic Equipment football helmet certification program. *Medicine and Science in Sports, 7*(3):225–232.

Hodgson VR (1980) Reducing Serious Injury in Sports. *Intrascholastic Athletic Association, 7*(2).

Jordan SE, Green GA, Galanty HL, et al. (1996) Acute and chronic brain injury in United States National Team Soccer Players. *The American Journal of Sports Medicine, 24*(2): 205–210.

Kaut KP, DePompei R, Kerr J, et al. (2003) Reports of head injury and symptom knowledge among college athletes: implications for assessment and educational intervention. *Clinical Journal of Sport Medicine, 12*, 213–221.

Kirkendall D, Jordan S, Garrett W (2001) Heading and head injuries in soccer. *Sports Medicine, 31*, 369–86.

Labella CR, Smith BW, Sigurdsson A (2002) Effect of mouthguards on dental injuries and concussions in college basketball. *Medicine and Science in Sports and Exercise, 34*(1): 41–44.

Levy ML, Ozgur BM, Berry C et al. (2004a) Analysis and evolution of head injury in football. *Neurosurgery, 55*, 649–655.

Levy ML, Ozgur BM, Berry C et al. (2004b) Birth and Evolution of the football helmet. *Neurosurgery, 55*, 656–662.

Lewis L, Naunheim RS, Standeven J et al. (2001) Do football helmets reduce acceleration of impact in blunt head injuries. *Academic Emergency Medicine, 8*, 604–609.

Lovell MR, Fazio V (2008) Concussion Management in the Child and Adolescent Athlete. *Current Sports Medicine Reports, 7*(1): 12–15.

McCaffrey MA, Mihalik JP, Crowell, DH et al. (2007) Measurement of Head Impacts in Collegiate Football Players: Clinical Measures of Concussion after High and Low Magnitude Impacts. *Neurosurgery, 61*, 1236–1243.

McCrea M, Hammeke T, Olsen G, et al. (2004) Unreported Concussion in high school football players; implication for prevention. *Clinical Journal of Sport Medicine, 14*(1): 13–17.

McCrory P, Collie A, Anderson V et al. (2004) Can we manage sport related concussion in children the same as in adults? *British Journal of Sports Medicine, 38*, 516–519.

McGuine T, Nass S (1996) Football Helmet Fitting Errors IN Wisconsin High School Players. Safety in American Football, American Society for Testing Materials 83–88.

McIntosh AS (2005) Risk compensation, motivation, injuries, and biomechanics in competitive sport. *British Journal of Sports Medicine, 39*, 2–3.

McIntosh AS, McCrory P (2000) Impact energy attenuation performance of football headgear. *British Journal of Sports Medicine, 34*, 337–341.

McIntosh AS, McCrory P (2005) Preventing head and neck injury. *British Journal of Sports Medicine, 39*, 314–318.

McIntosh AS, McCrory P, Comerford J (2000) The dynamics of concussive head impacts in rugby and Australian rules football. *Medicine and Science in Sports and Exercise, 32*(12): 1980–1984.

McIntosh AS, McCrory P, Finch CF (2004) Performance enhanced headgear: a scientific approach to the development of protective headgear. *British Journal of Sports Medicine, 38*, 46–49.

McIntosh AS, McCrory P, Finch CF, et al. (2009) Does Padded Headgear Prevent Head Injury in Rugby Union Football. *Medicine and Science in Sports and Exercise, 41*(2): 306–313.

Mihalik JP, Bell DR, Marshall SW et al. (2007) Measurement of Head Impacts in Collegiate Football Players: An Investigation of Positional and Event-Type Differences. *Neurosurgery, 61*, 1229–1235.

Naunheim RS, Standeven J, Richter C, et al. (2000) Comparison of impact data in hockey football, and soccer. *The Journal of Trauma, 48*, 938–941.

Naunheim R, McGurren M, Standeven J, et al. (2002) Does the use of artificial turf contribute to head injuries? *The Journal of Trauma, 53*, 691–694.

NOCSAE Standard Test Method and Equipment Used in Evaluating performance Characteristics of Protective Headgear /Equipment NOCSAE DOC (ND) 001-08m10 (2010) available at http://www.nocsae.org/standards/pdfs/Standards%20'10/ND001-08m10-Drop%20Impact%20Test%20Method%20.pdf accessed 3/24/11.

Pashby T, Carson JD, Ordogh D, et al. (2001) Eliminate head checking in ice hockey. *Clinical Journal of Sport Medicine, 11*, 211–213.

Pellman EJ (2003) Background on the NFL's research on concussion in professional football. *Neurosurgery, 53*, 797–798.

Pellman EJ, Viano DC, Tucker AM et al. (2003a) Concussion in Professional Football: Reconstruction of Game Impacts and Injuries. *Neurosurgery, 53*, 799–814.

Pellman EJ, Viano DC, Tucker AM et al. (2003b) Concussion in Professional Football: Location and direction of helmet impacts- Part 2. *Neurosurgery, 53*, 1328–1341.

Pellman EJ, Viano DC, Withnall C et al. (2006) Concussion in Professional Football: Helmet Testing to Assess Impact Performance- Part 11. *Neurosurgery, 58*, 78–96.

Putukian M, Echemendia RJ, Mackin S (2000) The Acute Neuropsychological Effects of Heading in Soccer: A Pilot Study. *Clinical Journal of Sport Medicine, 10*, 104–109.

Schnebel B, Gwin JT, Anderson S et al. (2007) In Vivo Study of Head Impacts in Football: A Comparison of National Collegiate Athletic Association Division I versus High School Impacts. *Neurosurgery, 60*, 490–496.

Singh GD, Maher GJ, Padilla RR (2009) Customized mandibular orthotics in the prevention of concussion/mild traumatic brain injury in football players: a preliminary study. *Dental Traumatology, 25*, 515–521.

Stuart MJ, Smith AM, Malo-Ortiguera SA, et al. (2002) A Comparison of Facial protection and the incidence of head, neck, and facial injuries in junior a hockey players. *The American Journal of Sports Medicine, 30*(1): 39–44.

Takeda T, Ishigami K, Hoshina S, et al. (2005) Can mouthguards prevent mandibular bone fracture and concussions? A laboratory study with an artificial skull model. *Dental Traumatology, 21,* 134–140.

Torg JS. The epidemiologic, biomechanical, and cinematographic analysis of football-induced cervical spine trauma and its prevention. In Torg JS (ed): *Athletic injuries to the head, neck, and face.* St Louis, Mosby-Year Book, 1991, 97–111.

Viano DC, Pellman EJ (2005) Concussion in Professional Football: Biomechanics of the Striking Player- Part 8. *Neurosurgery, 56,* 266–280.

Viano DC, Casson IR, Pellman EJ et al. (2005a) Concussion in Professional Football: Brain Responses by Finite Element Analysis: Part 9. *Neurosurgery, 57*(17): 891–916.

Viano DC, Casson IR, Pellman EJ et al. (2005b) Concussion in Professional Football: Comparison with Boxing Head Impacts- Part 10. *Neurosurgery, 57,* 1154–1172.

Viano DC, Pellman, EJ, Withnall C et al. (2006) Concussion in Professional Football: Performance of newer helmets in reconstructed game impacts-Part 13. *Neurosurgery, 59,* 591–606.

Viano DC, Casson IR, Pellman EJ (2007) Concussion in Professional Football: Biomechanics of the Struck Player- Part 14. *Neurosurgery, 61,* 313–328.

Wisniewski JF, Guskiewicz K, Trope M, et al. (2004) Incidence of cerebral concussions associated with type of mouthguard used in college football. *Dental Traumatology, 20,* 143–149.

Withnall C, Shewchenko N, Wonnacott M, et al. (2005) Effectiveness of headgear in football. *British Journal of Sports Medicine, 39,* (Suppl 1):i40–i48.

Chapter 14
Postinjury Issues and Ethics of Return to Play in Pediatric Concussion

Jennifer Niskala Apps, Kevin D. Walter, and Jason S. Doescher

14.1 Introduction

Throughout this book, an attempt has been made to consolidate, for the first time in one place, the limited but varied information available regarding the experience of concussion in children and adolescents. At this early developmental stage, it often seems that there are more questions than answers, which is true in any new medical area. As a result, at the publishing of this book a common complaint heard is that diagnosis of concussion is occurring at a much higher rate, but treatment options remain limited and long-term implications of the diagnosis are relatively unknown. Based on current research, how can a clinician best guide treatment? How can a parent make the best decisions for their child, particularly an adolescent for whom sports participation may have been at least a passion and at most his/her entire world, with some children relying on sports participation as a foundation for funding their future education?

J.N. Apps (✉)
Department of Psychiatry and Behavioral Medicine, Medical College of Wisconsin

Pediatric Neuropsychologist, Children's Hospital of Wisconsin, Milwaukee, WI, USA
e-mail: JApps@chw.org

K.D. Walter
Departments of Orthopaedics and Pediatrics, Medical College of Wisconsin

Program Director, Pediatric and Adolescent Sports Medicine, Children's Hospital of Wisconsin, Milwaukee, WI, USA

J.S. Doescher
Pediatric Neurology and Epilepsy, Minnesota Epilepsy Group, P.A.

Children's Hospital and Clinics of Minnesota, Saint Paul, MN, USA

J.N. Apps and K.D. Walter (eds.), *Pediatric and Adolescent Concussion: Diagnosis, Management and Outcomes*, DOI 10.1007/978-0-387-89545-1_14,
© Springer Science+Business Media, LLC 2012

14.2 The Reality of Long-Term Implications

The reality, based on research findings, of experiencing a concussion is that it increases that person's risk of sustaining another concussion. Further, concussions appear to have an exponential neurocognitive impact, resulting in longer recovery times and increased symptom expression with each concussion (Guskiewicz et al. 2003; Zemper 2003). However, this potential vulnerability to additional concussions and exponential expansion of symptoms with each additional injury are also individual. As has been mentioned in several places throughout this book, multiple different preexisting environmental, genetic, and psychosocial factors likely play a role in these differences. However, the current state of knowledge does not allow for an accurate estimation of a person's relative risk for injury.

As a result, there is no existing standard for how many concussions are too many or when treatment decisions should change from a focus on recovery with return to activity to avoidance of high-risk sport (McCrory 2011). Cantu recommends retirement is strongly considered for any athlete that has sustained three concussions in a single season or has had postconcussive symptoms for at least 3 months (Cantu 2009, 2003). Since this decision is so individual, but also so important, the American Academy of Pediatrics recommends that any clinician that is uncomfortable with making a determination about withholding a young athlete for a length of time or that is contemplating a recommendation of retirement refer the patient to a specialist with expertise in sport-related concussion (Halstead et al. 2010).

14.2.1 Possible Long-Term Neurological Complications Following Concussion

Regardless of the method of assessment for postconcussion symptoms, the monitoring and documentation of Postconcussion Syndrome (PCS) is an important component of long-term decision-making.

As mentioned elsewhere in this text, a significant number of postconcussive measures are now available for reporting and measuring neurobehavioral symptoms. While representative examples have been given of what postinjury rating scales may look like, an attempt to exhaustively cover the myriad of options was outside the scope of this work. Rather, many scales are inappropriately worded for children or adolescents or have so little empirical data supporting their use in pediatrics, their use is minimal. The development of age-appropriate measures providing reliability and validity data within these populations is ongoing and will be an important component of growth in this field in the near future.

Computerized measures are gaining widespread popularity due to convenience. The use of more traditional neuropsychological testing also remains an important component of long-term monitoring for PCS symptoms. However, the use of computerized testing and traditional neuropsychological testing has limited research data supporting long-term risk of play decisions based on the complexity or length of recovery time.

14.2.1.1 Chronic Traumatic Encephalopathy

Research has begun to demonstrate dramatic and frightening possibilities with regard to Chronic Traumatic Encephalopathy (CTE). Martland first called this "punch drunk" or dementia pugilistica in 1928. In 2009, McKee et al. found that repetitive concussion, and likely even exposure to repetitive head impacts is associated with the development of CTE. CTE is a progressive neurodegenerative disease that occurs years after recovery from the acute effects of head trauma. CTE often begins as a midlife personality change, with behavior and mood disturbance. Early signs and symptoms include irritability, anger and being hyper-emotional or "punchy". CTE appears to have a slow but progressive course. Advanced stage CTE has signs of dementia, Parkinsonism, speech and gait abnormalities, and it may be misdiagnosed as Alzheimer disease.

There have been cases of tau protein pathology, believed to correspond with CTE, reported in a high school football player and collegiate football players upon autopsy (McKee 2011). In 2005, Omalu et al. reported on the first known case of CTE in a National Football League (NFL) player, with the number of affected NFL players growing based on the work of Drs. Omalu and McKee (Omalu et al. 2010). However, CTE remains controversial, as it is difficult to prove a link between head trauma and tau pathology in the brain without improved prospective research (Casson 2010).

Apolipoprotein E (APOE) is an established genetic marker for Alzheimer disease (Kim et al. 2009). APOE may be associated with increased risk of concussion. Tierney et al. (2010) and Terrell et al. (2008) reported that APOE increased the likelihood of multiple concussions in collegiate male football and female soccer players. APOE appears to be associated with chronic traumatic brain injury in boxers (Jordan et al. 1997). However, there have not been any large studies and it is difficult to account for the multicausality of concussion as well as the individual variation in the manifestations of APOE (Teasdale et al. 1997; Gordon 2010). Thus, at this time there is not enough evidence to link APOE to concussion risk.

14.2.1.2 Headache

Further, while the frequency in children and adolescents is unclear, some individuals experience chronic headaches subsequent to a concussion. In 2008, Stovner et al. reported that the main risk factor of recurrent headache 3 months after a concussion was a history of pretraumatic headaches. A review of studies investigating TBI and chronic pain revealed posttraumatic headaches in nearly 58% of patients; however, this study was done using adults and more severe TBI (Nampiaparampil 2008). While some authors attribute posttraumatic headaches to psychological disorders and stress from litigation concerns, it also appears that analgesic overuse, particularly ibuprofen/NSAID rebound, is responsible for what appears to be posttraumatic headache (Warner and Fenichel 1996). It appears that posttraumatic headaches can be treated effectively using antimigraine therapy (Weiss et al. 1991). Headaches may also be treated with physical therapy and "alternative" therapies, such as acupuncture and chiropractic care. Again, more research is needed focused on the pediatric and adolescent population and the sport-related concussion population to identify the true incidence of posttraumatic headache and the best treatment options.

14.2.1.3 Seizure

Equally unclear is the experience of an increased seizure disorder risk following a head injury. While posttraumatic epilepsy (PTE) is a known complication of traumatic brain injury (TBI), the incidence is unclear. Increased severity of TBI is associated with increased risk of late, occurring greater than 1 week postinjury, seizures or epilepsy (Annegers and Coan 2000; Christensen et al. 2009; Ferguson et al. 2009). A family history of epilepsy notably increases the risk of PTE (Christensen et al. 2009). The reported overall incidence of PTE ranges from 13 to 50%, but studies have been completed using more severe TBI in adult and primarily military populations (Ferguson et al. 2009). Ferguson et al. found that severe TBI, history of depression and posttraumatic seizures prior to discharge were risk factors for PTE. Continued research needs to be done to clarify the risk of PTE in the young population and the risk of PTE from sport-related concussion.

14.2.2 Possible Long-Term Social and Emotional Complications Following Concussion

Aside from attempting to understand and balance the significant neurophysiological risks associated with a single versus multiple concussions, also discussed at length in various points throughout this book are the psychological, social and environmental impacts of these injuries. While formal data is clearly limited, it is evident that psychosocial factors play a key role prior to injury, interact significantly with the injury process and can have a significant impact on recovery. Consensus statements acknowledge that preexisting mental health issues, for example, can impact recovery from injury (McCrory et al. 2009), and the complexity of these interactions contributes to the difficulties quantifying and defining recovery.

From a subjective, clinical perspective, many adolescents with concussion experience significant difficulties with the nature of the recommendations for recovery. To remove an adolescent from social and athletic activities, for even a short period of time, often has a significant ramification for their social and emotional functioning. At a time in development when individuals are most clearly measured against their peers and establishing their unique identity, concussion management recommendations and restrictions can increase stress. This stress occurs with removal from the majority of peer interactions at school, team activities, and extra-curricular social situations. Limitations on electronic communications such as tex-ting and social communication can increase feelings of isolation. Further, concussion may prevent an adolescent from participating in social events such as homecoming or prom, as well as interfere with collegiate testing such as the ACT or SAT. Asking the adolescent to accept modifications in school can set them apart academically at a time when they are extremely sensitive to differences from others and may nega-tively impact their ability to self-advocate. Further, many athletically oriented teen-agers are also relatively goal-oriented, and their increased academic struggles, need for academic assistance and even problems on seminal academic testing that occurs at this age can cause legitimate anxiety about the impact such an injury could have on future academic plans.

A concussion's potentially complicated impact on life may increase the risk of social maladjustment or emotional reactivity in the teenager. Such reactions can further complicate the recovery process itself, as they quickly become confused with other PCS symptoms, such as increased irritability, depression, and anxiety. For a high-achieving junior in high school, with a prior strong academic record and plans for college attendance and athletics participation, recovery from a concussion lasting 3–4 months can severely impact their future. Without proper advocacy and education of the school and other individuals, the child can risk losing academic standing, which impacts college admission and ultimately their life goals. Add to these anxieties the loss of their usual active, athletic lifestyle, possibly their social support network of a team sports environment, and the frustration of other students, friends, teachers, and adults not understanding the realities of prolonged cognitive and neurophysiological recovery, and it is understandable what a significant impact such an injury can have.

Children and adolescents who were already struggling with mental health issues can exacerbate these issues. Children and adolescents who may have had a tendency toward anxiety or depression prior to injury may experience such an increase in stress as to become symptomatic for the first time. Further, symptoms of depression and anxiety can be symptomatic of the injury itself, resolving over time along with other symptoms. However, data regarding the confounding factors of emotional functioning at baseline (prior to injury) are limited. It is far more common to find research among larger TBI populations in general, adult, or geriatric populations, and even among military or veteran populations. The extrapolation of this to the pediatric population is limited at this time.

14.2.3   The Reality of Treatment Options

Aside from the "standard of care" – no one knows with certainty what else to do!!

Monitoring an individual's speed of symptom resolution remains one method of on-going assessment. Augmenting this monitoring with neurocognitive testing can be even more revealing. The use of computerized measures is gaining widespread popularity because of their significant strengths: ease of administration, ability to administer serial evaluations, ability to capture "baseline" data easily, and the convenience of providing such testing in a wide variety of settings without the need for specialized personnel. In addition to ImPACT testing, which has been thoroughly reviewed in this book as an excellent example of this type of product, there are other products including HeadMinder, CogState, and ANAM. HeadMinder is a company developed to utilize technology in cognitive assessment for a wide variety of diseases and injuries. They offer the Concussion Resolution Index, an Internet-based neurocognitive test measuring reaction time, memory, speeded decision-making, and neurophysiological symptoms of a concussion. CogState is a similar company providing cognitive testing across the globe. CogState Sport offers computerized concussion management software, which in North America is serviced through Axon Sports. They also offer an internet-based testing option, which allows for the sharing of test results electronically with a wide variety of providers and caregivers. The Automated Neuropsychological Assessment Metrics (ANAM) battery of computerized cognitive tests was developed for military use. Baseline testing is now a mandatory requirement prior to deployment.

However, the use of neurocognitive testing is also limited by preexisting cognitive issues, such as learning disabilities or attention disorders, as well as any confounding adjustment issues related to the injury itself. Baseline testing can present difficulties for interpretation as well, particularly in situations where children have decided to attempt to "trick the test" or not put forth adequate effort to purposefully lower their baseline scores, or have preexisting conditions that impact preinjury performances (Bailey et al. 2010). Such difficulties further the need for qualified neuropsychologists to complete more thorough cognitive evaluations when assessing long-term symptoms as a whole, rather than relying strictly on screening or computerized test results.

As medical personnel or parents, our goal is to utilize incoming information to determine an appropriate treatment plan. Regardless of the pressures to return quickly to athletics or other activities, at times the correct treatment approach is prolonged removal from activity. At this stage of knowledge, even high-level athletes are making significant career decisions based on limited understanding of the long-term risks of concussion recovery. If these athletes can make career decisions out of concern for their future cognitive health, the relative importance of a few high school games should be viewed in perspective. However, by contrast, treatment planning also needs to acknowledge and encourage the child or adolescent to gradually return to normal activity levels. Particularly in cases of prolonged symptoms, it can become intimidating and overwhelming to return to physical activity or academic and cognitive tasks. An important component of the treatment plan needs to be clear and explicit assistance in helping that child and their parents in developing slow, steady progression that is not stressful to the point of exacerbating symptoms due to increased anxiety and emotional reactivity.

14.2.3.1 Active Rehabilitation

There is emerging evidence that "active rehabilitation" from concussion may be helpful. Much of this focuses on subsymptom threshold exercise training in patients with postconcussion syndrome (PCS). In 2010, Leddy et al. showed that adult PCS patients that performed controlled aerobic exercise 5–6 days per week had greater improvement in PCS symptoms compared to PCS patients that continued to rest. The patient was exerted using a reliable, graded treadmill test to identify a heart rate that consistently exacerbated symptoms (Leddy et al. 2011). Exercise was performed at 80% of that heart rate, thus subsymptom threshold training. Athletes perceive exercise as a positive activity, which can immediately decrease symptoms of depression.

A small study done on children 10–17 years of age with over 4 weeks of concussion symptoms showed benefits of active rehabilitation (Gagnon et al. 2009). All of these children were initially felt to be recovering slowly when they were enrolled in a closely monitored active rehabilitation program involving 50–60% max capacity aerobic activity for up to 15 min, but stopping earlier if they developed symptoms. Also included were coordination exercises and sports-related visualization activities. When these were done daily, all participants had a full recovery, with most taking less than 1 month to return. These emerging positive benefits herald the need for further research into this promising intervention.

14.2.3.2 Vestibular Rehabilitation

Vestibular rehabilitation is gaining acceptance in treatment of concussion. The vestibular system is our body's way of detecting linear and angular acceleration, and our perceived body orientation in space. The vestibular system helps coordinate postural stability (head, eye, and trunk movements) and also stabilizes our gaze or vision. Concussion can cause significant dizziness, loss of balance, and visual changes (double vision, blurry vision) that may be a result of vestibular dysfunction. Americans first used vestibular therapy for brain-injured soldiers in the mid-twentieth century (Cifu DX et al. 2010). Vestibular therapy can be used to help decrease dizziness and improve gait and balance. While vestibular therapy is usually quite individualized, frequently exercises are composed of gaze stabilization activities, standing balance activities, and walking balance maneuvers. Most patients, both children and adults, that underwent vestibular therapy reported improvement in their balance and dizziness symptoms (Alsalaheen et al. 2010). Research must continue to confirm the efficacy of vestibular therapy in the pediatric population and to understand the best timing for referral to a vestibular therapist (immediately or a few weeks postinjury).

14.2.3.3   Other Therapies

There is preliminary evidence that omega-3 fatty acid supplementation may be beneficial for head injury. In 2010, Bailes and Mills reported that docosahexaenoic acid (DHA) supplementation for 30 days after a head injury reduced axon damage. This may be due to a reduction in the inflammatory response of the body. Most omega-3 supplements are over the counter fish oil capsules and are not regulated by the Food and Drug Administration (FDA). Thus, companies may make claims that their supplements can decrease concussion risk and hasten concussion healing. These claims have no scientific basis. Further investigation is needed to show any benefit during the inflammatory phase of concussion.

In any evolving field in medicine, there will be many proposed new treatments that are unproven and may or may not end up being helpful. Concussion is no different, and in the coming years there will likely be many of these "treatments". For example, there have been anecdotal claims that hyperbaric oxygen therapy helps accelerate concussion healing. There is no proof that this is true. As a provider, it is important to consider the physiologic logic behind each proposed treatment, as well as the cost–benefit for any potential therapy. It is also paramount that the underlying principle of returning to play only when asymptomatic and after having received medical clearance is followed. Young athletes in particular may feel that a new "treatment" may make it safe for them to return to play earlier.

14.3   The Reality of Return to Play Decisions

With such a confusing complexity of risks, how do parents and professionals make return to play decisions that will respect the child or adolescent while offering them appropriate protection? The reality is that the current status of research supports only the use of return to play decisions thoroughly outlined in this book, based on the Zurich guidelines and adopted by position statements across organizations. It is important to remember that all return to play guidelines are mainly expert opinion and not evidence-based. However, that should not deter the provider from utilizing the guidelines, as there is much to be gained from the insight of experts in the field that have cared for concussion. Little to no information is available on how to manage or consider the extensive psychosocial impact of the injury, prolonged recovery, or the question of not returning to play (i.e., mandatory retirement from contact sports and high risk sports). When discussing retirement from activities, it is important to consider that a child that enjoys basketball can still shoot and play noncontact games such as "horse", but they should avoid competitive, rough, and organized basketball (Tables 14.1 and 14.2).

Rather, practitioners must utilize their clinical judgment and common sense in providing guidance and recommendations to families. Education to each patient and family is essential, as they all need to know that hiding or minimizing symptoms can have alarming consequences: postconcussion syndrome, second impact

Table 14.1 Examples of contact sports

- Football
- Soccer
- Ice Hockey
- Basketball
- Lacrosse
- Wrestling
- Sparring in martial arts
- Rugby
- Boxing

Table 14.2 Examples of high-risk sports

- Alpine sports (snowboarding, downhill skiing)
- Bicycle and BMX
- Diving
- Motor vehicle racing
- Skateboarding and scooter riding

syndrome, repeat injury, etc. Utilizing balance and neurocognitive tests as a tool can potentially improve safety when providing return to play guidance. However, it is imperative to understand that neuropsychological testing cannot stand alone in the decision-making process. Therefore, a young athlete may score at their baseline on a computerized test, but because he/she is still symptomatic, they are not qualified to begin a return-to-activity plan.

There are many patients that should not return to play using the standard Zurich guidelines (McCrory et al. 2009). This group includes patients with prolonged symptoms (arguably over 2–4 weeks), very severe symptoms, multiple concussions (2+) and those with comorbidities such as chronic headaches or mental health disorders. This can be very subjective criteria, and utilization often depends on the comfort level and experience of each treating provider. A provider experienced in management of concussion and postconcussion syndrome should ideally treat this group of patients. These patients require substantial education regarding their increased risk of repeat concussion, consideration for retirement or substantial time away from contact sports and high-risk activity and an extended, carefully monitored return to play protocol. Patients that are difficult to treat due to poor compliance, erratic behavior, or other social concerns should also receive consideration for more slow or conservative return to activity plans.

In discussing retirement, it is the authors' opinion that it is imperative to follow "trends" in patients with multiple concussions. For example, if each subsequent concussion is caused by a lesser force, that is a concerning trend. It is concerning when each subsequent concussion lasts longer or has more intense symptoms. Another concerning trend is when concussions begin to occur quickly or with increasing frequency. If a provider can identify these trends in a young athlete, it is reasonable to begin restrictions and retirement earlier to prevent potential long-term postconcussion syndrome or chronic/permanent adverse sequelae.

Another ethical concern that must be considered regarding young athletes is the motivation to return. It is essential not to treat a scholarship or high-level athlete with aspirations to play professionally any differently than a recreational athlete. Most professional athletes have very short athletic careers and will need full cognitive function to become productive members of society after they retire from sports.

Some young athletes will have tremendous external pressure placed on them to return to play. Providers should be able to identify the origin of the pressure to eliminate or decrease it. Pressure can come from a coach pushing to get his starting player back into the game. Unfortunately even at the youth and high school levels, coaches are judged based on their win–loss record, and they need to continue to win to keep their jobs. This can create a conflict of interest for even the most well-intentioned coach. Coaches and parents often have misconceptions of concussion management, often referencing how they were "treated" in their youth. Education goes a long way in detailing how knowledge of the injury and treatment have dramatically improved over the last decade. Parents may also pressure their child to get back into the game for fear of missing out on a scholarship. Some parents push their child aggressively to accomplish athletic goals that they could not accomplish in their youth. It is also reasonable to consider that families have significant amounts of money wrapped up in athletics, and helping the family recoup any potential money due to missed time may be helpful.

Finally, some athletes pressure themselves to return. Often young athletes use their sport as their identity. If they are held out of activity, they lose that sense of identity. Athletes also do not want to be perceived as "wimpy" or "soft" by their peers and teammates because they are missing time due to an injury. Complicating this feeling is that the athlete often looks "normal" because concussion is an injury that does not require a cast or a brace that serves as a visual reminder of the injury. Adequate education of the athlete, team, and coaching staff can help reduce that tension. On the other side, athletes may feel that an injury is the only way out of their sport. Young athletes may feel forced to participate in a sport by peers and parents, when they have no interest in playing. These young athletes will complain of persistent symptoms to remain on the sideline. Often, they will not have any problems in the classroom or with "screen time" (TV, computer, video games, etc.), but still complain of symptoms that would likely cause problems in those arenas. In these cases, providers should carefully navigate the rationale for participation from the athlete and his/her parents, and offer alternatives to participation, such as becoming the manager, using practice time to volunteer, or joining another sport or extracurricular activity.

14.3.1 Legal Mandates on Return to Play

In 2009, Washington passed the Lystedt Law, becoming the first state to legislate protection for young athletes with concussion (Washington House Bill 1824). This law was named after Zackery Lystedt, a 13-year-old young athlete that was permanently disabled when he prematurely returned to play with a concussion. The law focuses on concussion education for anyone involved with young athletes and not allowing a concussed athlete to return to play on the same day and without clearance from an appropriate health-care provider. Since that time, similar legislation has been passed in many states. The primary focus is on education and awareness, as well as the mandate of no return to play on the same day as a concussion, no return to play with symptoms, and that all concussions need medical clearance prior to return to play. The definition of an appropriate health-care provider is unique to each state. Ideally, research will be done in states with concussion laws to assess for effectiveness in reducing complications of concussion and improving concussion management.

Nationally, there have been Congressional hearings regarding concussion from the youth level to the NFL. There is potential federal legislation for concussion (HR 1347) that is similar to state level legislation.

14.4   Conclusions

Now more than ever, better recognition exists of the neurocognitive effects of concussion. The complexities of this injury can be acknowledged, particularly during childhood and adolescence. All aspects of daily functioning are impacted by an injury that is not physically obvious, such as a broken leg treated in a cast. Social, emotional, and academic complications are all common. These complexities often confuse those who care about the child, allowing for an early return to prior activity levels to "get back to normal". However, increased understanding of the risks of reinjury and additional injury also provide more reasons to keep children out of activities.

Most of all, these clinical decisions impact the lives of a child and their family, possibly altering life goals and expectations. Life goals, college and career plans, and possible scholarships are all important life decisions being made at this time. Unfortunately, parents and children commonly need to advocate for their own recovery process with academic, athletic and occupational personnel that are under-educated and unaware of the impact of concussion. In severe cases, parents and teens may be asked to weigh options that include the loss of those future goals or possibilities versus the likelihood for long-term cognitive problems resulting from continued participation in high-risk sport and repeat injuries.

Increased awareness and education regarding recognition of concussion and the recovery process are integral to helping protect our children. Advocacy is an important component. Concussion education should be mandatory for all athletes, parents, and coaches involved in youth and high school athletics. Even further, there must be education for teachers, counselors and those working with children to help them understand how concussion adversely impacts the cognitive and functional abilities of a young person. These positive changes will only occur with advocacy at the local (community and school district), state, and national levels.

As awareness of concussions continues to increase, the focus on medical education and improved research will increase as well. Without an increase in research specifically focused on pediatric concussion, the ability to refine management guidelines will remain limited. As is obvious from the research highlighted by this book, much of what is known or assumed about pediatric concussion is extrapolated from adult studies, studies of children and adolescents with more severe traumatic brain injuries, or smaller studies with limited data. Only by increasing research funding and the specific study of concussion in children and adolescents will true advancements occur in understanding, preventing, and treating this injury. With increased awareness comes increased need for clinical care. With increased need for clinical care comes an increased need for greater understanding of the issues raised in this book.

14.5   Key Points

Research demonstrates that experiencing a concussion increases a person's risk of sustaining another concussion, causes exponential neurocognitive impact, and can result in longer recovery times and increased symptom expression.

No standards exist for how many concussions are too many.

Possible long-term neurological complications of concussion can include chronic traumatic encephalopathy, headaches, and seizure, although these occurrences are rare and poorly understood in children and adolescents at this time.

Psychosocial complications interact with concussion symptoms and recovery plans, often exacerbating physiological stress and emotional symptoms such as anxiety and depression.

Adolescents may require significant academic advocacy and educational efforts not to experience negative impacts on their academic future as a result of their concussion recovery.

Return to play decisions are ethically and medically complicated. Legal mandates will likely soon play a role in family's decision-making processes, but regardless of this, consultation with a professional experienced in management of youth concussion is strongly recommended.

References

Alsalaheen, B. A., Mucha, A., Morris, L. O., et al. (2010). Vestibular rehabilitation for dizziness and balance disorders after concussion. *Journal of Neurologic Physical Therapy, 34*, 87–93.

Annegers, J. F., & Coan, S. P. (2000). The risks of epilepsy after traumatic brain injury. *Seizure, 9*, 453–457.

Bailes, J. E., & Mills, J. D. (2010). Docosahexaenoic acid reduces traumatic axonal injury in a rodent head injury model. *Journal of Neurotrauma, 27*, 1617–1624.

Bailey, C. M., Samples, H. L., Broschek D. K., et al. (2010). The relationship between psychological distress and baseline sports-related concussion testing. *Clinical Journal of Sport Medicine, 20*(4), 272–277.

Casson IR. Do the 'facts' really support an association between NFL players' concussions, dementia and depression? Neurology Today 2010; June: 6–7.

Cantu, R. C. (2009). When to disqualify an athlete after a concussion. *Current Sports Medicine Reports, 8*(1), 6–7.

Cantu, R. C. (2003). Recurrent athletic head injury risks and when to retire. *Clinics in Sports Medicine, 22*(3), 593–603.

Christensen, J., Pedersen, M. G., Pederen, C. B., et al. (2009). Long-term risk of epilepsy after traumatic brain injury in children and young adults: a population-based cohort study. *The Lancet, 373*, 1105–1110.

Cifu, D. X., Cohen, S. I., Lew, H. L., et al. (2010). The history and evolution of traumatic brain injury rehabilitation in military service members and veterans. *American Journal of Physical Medicine and Rehabilitation, 89*, 688–694.

Ferguson, P. L., Smith, G. M., Wannamake, B. B., et al. (2009). A population-based study of the risk of epilepsy after hospitalization for traumatic brain injury. *Epilepsia, 51*, 891–898.

Gagnon, I., Galli, C., Friedman, D., et al. (2009). Active rehabilitation for children who are slow to recover following sport-related concussion. *Brain Injury, 23*, 956–964.

Gordon, K. E., & Apolipoprotein, E. (2010). Apolipoprotein E genotyping and concussion: time to fish or cut bait. *Clinical Journal of Sport Medicine, 20*, 405–6.

Guskiewicz, K., McCrea, M., Marshall, S., et al. (2003). Cumulative effects associated with recurrent concussion in collegiate football players. *JAMA, 290*, 2549–2555.

Halstead, M. E., Walter, K. D., et al. (2010). Clinical report – sport-related concussion in children and adolescents. *Pediatrics, 126*, 597–615.

Jordan, B. D., Relkin, N. R., Ravdin, L. D., et al. (1997). Apolipoprotein E epsilon 4 associated with chronic traumatic brain injury in boxing. *JAMA, 278*(2), 136–140.

Kim, J., Basak, J. M., & Holtzman, D. M. (2009). The role of apolipoprotein E in Alzheimer's disease. *Neuron, 63*, 287–303.

Leddy, J. J., Baker, J. G., Kozlowski, K., et al. (2011). Reliability of a graded exercise test for assessing recovery from concussion. *Clinical Journal of Sport Medicine, 21*, 89–94.

Leddy, J. J., Kozlowski, K., Donnelly, J., et al. (2010). A preliminary study of subsymptom threshold exercise training for refractory post-concussion syndrome. *Clinical Journal of Sport Medicine, 20*, 21–27.

Martland, H. S. (1928). Punch drunk. *JAMA, 91*, 1103–1107.

McCrory, P. (2011). When to retire after concussion? *British Journal of Sports Medicine, 45*(6), 380–382.

McCrory, P., Meeuwisse, W., Johnston, K., et al. (2009). Consensus statement on concussion in sport: The 3 rd International Conference on Concussion in Sport held in Zurich, November 2008. *British Journal of Sports Medicine, 43*(Suppl 1), 76–84.

McKee, A., Cantu, R., Nowinski, C., et al. (2009). Chronic traumatic encephalopathy in athletes: progressive tauopathy after repetitive head injury. *Journal of Neuropathology and Experimental Neurology, 68*, 709–735.

McKee AC. Chronic traumatic encephalopathy and chronic traumatic encephalomyelopathy. Presented at the 2011 University of Wisconsin Sports Medicine Symposium, April 7, 2011.

Nampiaparampil, D. E. (2008). Prevalence of chronic pain after traumatic brain injury. *JAMA, 300*, 711–719.

Omalu, B. I., DeKosky, S. T., Minster, R. L., et al. (2005). Chronic traumatic encephalopathy in a National Football League player. *Neurosurgery, 57*(1), 128–134.

Omalu, B. I., Hamilton, R. L., Kamboch, M. I., et al. (2010). Chronic traumatic encephalopathy in a national football league player: case report and emerging medicolegal practice questions. *Journal of Forensic Nursing, 6*, 40–46.

Stovner, L. J., Schrader, H., Mickeviciene, D., et al. (2008). Headache after concussion. *European Journal of Neurology, 16*, 112–120.

Teasdale, G. M., Nicoll, J. A., Murray, G., et al. (1997). Association of apolipoprotein E polymorphism with outcome after head injury. *The Lancet, 350*, 1069–1071.

Terrell, T. R., Bostick, R. M., Abramson, R., et al. (2008). APOE, APOE promoter, and tau genotypes and risk for concussion in college athletes. *Clinical Journal of Sport Medicine, 18*, 10–17.

Tierney, R., Mansell, J. L., Higgins, M., et al. (2010). APOE genotype and concussion in college athletes. *Clinical Journal of Sport Medicine, 20*, 464–468.

Warner, J. S., & Fenichel, G. M. (1996). Chronic post-traumatic headache often a myth? *Neurology, 46*, 915–916.

Weiss, H. D., Stern, B. J., & Goldberg, J. (1991). Post-traumatic migraine: chronic migraine precipitated by minor head or neck trauma. *Headache, 31*, 451–456.

Zemper, E. D. (2003). Two-year prospective study or relative risk of a second cerebral concussion. *American Journal of Physical Medicine & Rehabilitation, 82*(9), 653–659.

Index

J.N. Apps and K.D. Walter, *Pediatric and Adolescent Concussion:*
Diagnosis, Management and Outcomes, DOI 10.1007/978-0-387-89545-1,
© Springer Science+Business Media, LLC 2012

Printed by Publishers' Graphics LLC USA
MO20120330-02
2012